The Giving

stories of organ donation

with one small gesture
you can change someone's life

JK Bovi

---Dedications---

My liver donor and donor family
October 5, 2019

---Acknowledgments---

My husband Bob and my sister Pat
Sons Christopher and Robert
Daughter-in-law Julie
Friends and family

My Care Team - Mayo Clinic, Jacksonville, Florida
Liver Transplant Program
Critical Care Unit
Pulmonary Medicine

If this book helps one person, then it is enough.

Chapter One

The two sisters stood arm-in-arm in front of the weathered old beach house. The younger one leaned heavily on the older sibling. It's how they'd been all their lives, Patricia taking care of JoAnn.

"What do you think of the house rental?" Patricia asked.

"I think it's perfect."

"It's all I could find with such short notice and it being off-season and all that."

"I like it. It's just fine. Thank you for finding a place."

"It's on the ocean block. It's a short walk to the beach. When you're feeling better, we can walk there."

"That would be nice. I'd enjoy that." JoAnn forced a smile, but it couldn't be seen because of the white surgical mask covering her nose and mouth.

The pain from getting out of the rental car and standing in the driveway made her feel nauseous and weak. She wanted desperately to rest. Even the cracked cement driveway and dirt-covered front lawn looked like an inviting place to lay down.

Patricia sensed her sister's discomfort. "Let's go inside. You can rest." She spoke like someone who was used to being in charge.

Patricia had owned her own insurance business and, at the age of 55, sold it for a sizable amount. She was able to take an early retirement to do whatever she wanted and to go wherever she wished. She had traveled around Europe, took Caribbean cruises, and toured the Australian outback. It hadn't been part of her retirement plan to take care of JoAnn, but nobody expected her sister to need a liver transplant.

As predictable, Patricia flew down from Vermont in the middle of a snowstorm to get to the Mayo Clinic in Jacksonville, Florida to be at her sister's side for surgery and recovery.

JoAnn's voice was weak and had a tremble to it. "Yes. I would like to go inside and lie down."

Patricia led JoAnn to the front porch and, as they got closer, she was reminded how shoddy and dilapidated the rental truly was. She should've looked for something better. Her sister deserved more.

JoAnn was used to special treatment. She was two years younger than Patricia and had been coddled when they were children. Her husband had pampered her like a princess. They divorced when her neediness became a burden and he replaced her with a more accommodating wife. JoAnn didn't care about her failed marriage because they'd grown apart. Her husband, Carl, a corporate executive, kept their expensive home outside of Atlanta and she took the waterfront condo at Lake Lanier. He was a perfect southern gentleman and paid her alimony and covered her health insurance without complaint.

"Lean on me and I'll help you," Patricia said. They took the four steps up together and walked six steps to the front door. Patricia turned the tarnished brass doorknob to open the warped wooden door. "One more step up, and then we're in. Can you do one more step?"

JoAnn nodded and lifted her foot to place it on the step. The board creaked. She let Patricia guide her to a bedroom at the back of the house, but she could barely understand the words her sister spoke.

"This room is the smaller of the two, but it's close to the bathroom. It gets the afternoon sun, so you can sleep late. I'm in the next room. Here lay down."

JoAnn laid down on the soft bed, removed the mask from her face, crossed her arms over her chest, closed her eyes, and sighed with relief.

"Do you need anything?" Patricia asked.

"What?"

"Do you need anything?"

"No. No, thank you. I'm fine."

"Get some rest. I'll check on you in a little while." Patricia gently shut the door and gave out a sigh of relief of her own.

* * *

Patricia went into the kitchen to give it a good cleaning because, not only did it have outdated fixtures and appliances, it was dirty. Someone had made a feeble attempt to clean the laminated counters, wooden kitchen table, and the four chairs, but the toaster oven, stove, and refrigerator were in need of a good scrubbing. At least the microwave and coffee maker were new.

Because JoAnn had a liver transplant only four days ago and was released from the hospital, she had a compromised immune system. Any bad germs could cause an infection that could be life-threatening. As a caregiver, it was Patricia's job to make sure her sister was given time to heal in a germ-free environment.

The kitchen in the old beach house was definitely not clean, but after two hours of washing and scrubbing, Patricia had it sparkling like a Mister Clean TV advertisement. She made herself and JoAnn a healthy high-protein lunch of yogurt, salad, apple, and toast. She was careful to wash the lettuce, cucumber, tomatoes, and apple as instructed by the nutritionist.

She knocked on her sister's bedroom door but didn't get an answer. She opened the door and walked to the bed. JoAnn was just as she'd left her; on her back, arms crossed on her chest, and eyes closed. Patricia leaned in close to make sure she was breathing and not dead. Having her sister die on her watch would be a horrible thing.

"JoAnn wake up. I made us some lunch."

JoAnn opened her eyes and smiled. "Oh, thank you. I am hungry," she said and attempted to get up herself, but she was unsure how to move correctly because of her abdominal stitches. Patricia helped her to sit on the edge of the bed. From there they went to the bathroom and JoAnn said she could take care of herself, but Patricia hovered outside the closed door and waited. She heard her sister say, "This stitch is for love, this one for gratitude, this is to say thank you, and this reminds me to be strong for my donor, and this one is a thank you for my gift of life."

JoAnn opened the door and smiled. "I'm ready for some lunch, but after that, I'd like to sit on the porch swing, if that's okay."

"It's okay with me. Of course, the swing is so old, the chains could break and you might fall on your butt."

They laughed together, and then JoAnn said, "There are no guarantees in life."

The butterfly counts not months
but moments, and has time enough.

--Rabindranath Tagore

Chapter Two

The beach house wasn't located on a secluded quiet beach but instead wedged between two other rental properties on a narrow beach block street in Neptune Beach, Florida. A fence surrounded the backyard for privacy.

The house on the left was a towering pristine two-story white building with turquoise trim around the windows and the porch railings. It looked fun and inviting for renters staying upstairs and downstairs. The little cottage on the right was brightly painted yellow with purple trim and decorated with plastic fish, seashells, and rubber crabs.

Their beach rental was a paint chipped shingled single-story house. A broken ceramic vase lay in the dirt in the front yard, two stone pillars were at each corner of the property with cracked old flower pots adorning the tops. On the porch, dangling on rusty chains, hung a wooden two-seater swing. Next to the swing was a rusty metal table, a wooden chair and a matching rocking chair. Everything was ugly, dismal and uninviting.

Attached to the house was a single-car garage and above the garage was an apartment. To get upstairs a person needed to use the door to the stairs between the house and the garage. This was where the landlord's son, Rick lived. He had shown Patricia the inside of the house and agreed to let her sign a month's contract. When he heard about JoAnn's liver transplant, he gave them a 10 % discount.

Rick was a good-looking 23-year-old man with a tan, sun-blonde hair, and a physique that would turn any young girl's head. He was a graduate of the University of Florida. He spent his days surfing and his nights bartending at his father's bar, The Alley Cat.

Rick bounded down the narrow steps, swung open the door, let it slam shut, and was about to head for the beach when he noticed the woman seated on the porch swing. He adjusted the surfboard under his arm and approached to introduce himself. "Hello. You must be Patricia's sister."

JoAnn had been shaken awake by the loud slam of the apartment door. She sat bundled up in a big fluffy sweater, baggie jogging pants, thick socks, fuzzy pink slippers, and a huge thick blanket. Her ensemble was accented by a wool hat on her head. Although it was February and it should be warm, it was chilly. She smiled pleasantly but inside, she was frowning, wondering if people would ever stop referring to her as *'Patricia's sister'*.

"Yes. I'm JoAnn. You must be Rick."

He stopped at the edge of the porch and ventured to take a step up. "So, how's the new liver doing?"

"I feel good today. Thank you for asking."

"They do a good job over there at Mayo. You'll be better in no time at all."

"I'm sure I'll be just fine, but I'm a bit worried about you. Isn't it rather cold to be out surfing?"

Rick, dressed in his sleek black wet suit laughed. "No worries. This wet suit will keep me warm enough to catch a few waves."

"What about sharks? Aren't there sharks out there?"

Rick was moved by her sincere concern. The only woman in his life who cared about him was his grandmother. She lived on the West Coast and called him once a week to chat. "All the sharks went to warmer waters in the Caribbean. Lots of tourists there for them to chomp on."

They laughed and JoAnn said, "Thanks for the laugh. Laughter is the best medicine."

"And good for the soul."

She nodded in agreement.

Rick thought she seemed a bit tired and that he should let her get back to her nap. "I better get on my way. Surfs up!"

"Be careful. Don't make me have to come looking for you!"

He laughed and waved goodbye.

* * *

JoAnn closed her eyes and, if she tried hard enough, she could hear the distant ocean waves, but it sounded more like a woman's soft sorrowful voice. The voice said, *'Change the baby'*. The voice repeated the words over and over until JoAnn fell asleep.

Patricia woke JoAnn with a gentle tap on her shoulder. She'd been shopping and carried a box containing a plastic shower chair that she'd have to put together. "I got a shower chair so you can sit in the shower. I also got a scale and a blood pressure cuff because I'm supposed to monitor your weight and blood pressure twice a day."

Patricia dashed into the house, and then returned to the car for the other items. Her last bag was full of groceries. "Are you hungry?"

"No, not really."

"You have to eat something."

"Yeah, okay."

"And you need to take your pills."

"Do I have any appointments today?"

"No. Blood work tomorrow morning, then meeting with Doctor Kennedy. Today you can rest. It's Sunday."

"Oh, is it? That's nice."

Patricia went into the house and left the front door open with the screen door closed. JoAnn could hear her talking about something to do with people at the grocery store and what she was making for lunch.

JoAnn felt someone sit on the swing beside her and looked to see who it was. The pretty young woman in the flowered sundress, with long blonde hair and a freckled nose was seated beside her. The woman smiled and said, *'Change the baby'*.

JoAnn jerked from what she thought was a dream but realized she wasn't asleep and the vision of the young woman could've been real! She quickly looked around the porch but saw no one nearby. She shivered, forced herself to stand up and walk into the house to the safety of the small kitchen.

Patricia rushed to her. "What's wrong? You, okay? You look pale and you're shaking. You look like you've seen a ghost or something?"

JoAnn sat at the table and said, "I'm fine. What's for lunch?" She decided that tomorrow she'd ask Doctor Kennedy at Mayo if any of the medications she was on caused hallucinations. The young woman on the porch swing had seemed unnervingly real.

Every day may not be good
But there's something good in every day.

--Alice Morse Earle

Chapter Three

Patricia woke to the voices of two people yelling at each other in the driveway. It was two o'clock in the morning! She recognized Rick's voice saying, "It's only for a month. Why are you so upset?"

An angry man yelled, "I told you I didn't want to rent this out!"

"It's extra money. We can use the money to fix this place up."

"I don't want to fix it up. I want it to stay how it is. I want it left alone. Why couldn't you do that? Why did you have to open this place up?"

"Come on Dad. We pay taxes on it, pay all the utilities, and get nothing. It should be profitable."

"I don't care about the money. It was bad enough when you decided to move into the apartment and now you want to rent out the house too? I told you no. No means no. What don't you understand?"

Patricia pulled on her bathrobe and peeked in JoAnn's room to be certain she was asleep, then she hurried across the living room, swung open the front door, and stomped down the steps to confront Rick and the man he was yelling at. "Can you two please keep your voices down? My sister is sleeping. She needs her rest. She's just had a liver transplant."

The man glared at her with annoyance, then he frowned at Rick.

Rick ignored his father's angry stare and smiled at Patricia. "I'm sorry. We didn't mean to wake you. This is my father, Bill." He then said to his father, "Dad, this is our renter, Patricia. Her sister is JoAnn and they'll only be here for a month."

"Yeah. Well, that's a month too long." He looked directly at Patricia with a not-to-friendly glare. "Find another place to stay."

"We can't do that. I can't move my sister all over the place. She's immune-compromised and could die. Then how would you feel about that?"

Bill clenched his teeth. He was in his late 50s, and when he wasn't yelling, he was good-looking, but at this moment he had no intention of being nice. "Not my problem. Get out of my house. Find another place to stay." He turned sharply, got into his car, and called out the window to his son, "I want them out!" He backed out of the driveway and drove away.

Patricia hugged her bathrobe around herself and looked at Rick. "Do we have to move out?"

"No. Dad will calm down. He's just a bit stubborn and obsessed with this house. He lived here with my mom, but when she died, he closed it up and walked away."

Patricia didn't like Bill causing trouble. She had dealt with trouble all her business life and now she wanted her life to be peaceful. "Maybe I can talk with him."

Rick shrugged his shoulders. "I wouldn't bother. He'll settle down."

She remembered Rick telling her his father owned a bar in town called The Alley Cat. Tomorrow she'd stop by so they could fight it out like a couple of alley cats.

The wings of transformation are
born of patience and struggle.

--Janet Dickens

Chapter Four

JoAnn sat patiently in the office waiting for Dr. Kennedy. She'd read over the postings on the wall three times and had studied the plastic model of a healthy liver. She had been gifted a new strong liver because her liver had been scarred and damaged by a rare disease: Autoimmune Hepatitis. Her liver disease was an unusual genetic condition that caused her immune system to think her liver was a foreign object and attacked it to the point that it was scarred, barely working, and dried up like a prune.

She'd been able to control her disease for five years with medications, but as time went on, her liver began failing and she reached stage 4 cirrhosis. Most people thought she was a *'closet alcoholic'*, but she only drank on special occasions. She gave up trying to convince people otherwise. They could think whatever they wanted, she no longer cared.

Her ex-husband, Carl, had been with her at her diagnosis and was sympathetic to her plight, but as time went by, he lost interest and she struggled alone. Her two children, Beth (18), and Jacob (25), were concerned but assumed their mother was strong enough to get through her physical problems without them being overly involved. Beth and Jacob called weekly to keep her updated on what they were doing, but JoAnn kept the details of her illness to herself.

Beth was a freshman at Valdosta State University studying psychology. JoAnn didn't know what a person could do with a bachelor's degree in psychology except maybe psychoanalyze their friends. No matter what she thought, she wholeheartedly supported her daughter's choice.

Jacob had received his law degree from Emory University and was studying for the Georgia bar exam. He had married a nice woman from Charleston South Carolina and soon, they'd have a baby. JoAnn was looking forward to being a grandmother and buying baby shoes, and clothes. She liked to decorate rooms and hoped they'd ask her to decorate the baby's room. She wanted to spend time just hugging and spoiling the little one. She wasn't overly excited about changing soiled diapers and she'd need to avoid that!

The door opened, and Dr. Kennedy stepped in with Andrea, the post-transplant coordinator. They shook hands with JoAnn and Patricia. Dr. Kennedy immediately sat down at the desktop computer to turn it on. He was a good-looking serious man with an Irish accent and he was *'all-business'*. He had been her hepatologist from when she first visited Mayo Clinic. He was familiar with her health issues and had guided her through the transplant process.

He looked at the numbers from her morning lab report, then turned in his chair, smiled, and said, "Everything looks good. How are you feeling?"

"Good."

"Good. Keep moving and take your medication."

JoAnn nodded in obedience. She got on the exam table as instructed and Andrea checked her blood pressure with the gauge, then Dr. Kennedy pressed here and there around her abdomen to check things out and studied her line of staples. She sat upright. Using his stethoscope, he listened to her heart, then he put the stethoscope to her chest and listened as she breathed in and out. When finished with the exam, she sat down beside her sister.

Dr. Kennedy returned to his desk. "Everything looks fine. The numbers are great. Are you having any problems with the medications?"

JoAnn didn't know about the medications. There were too many for her to remember and she had no idea what their names were or the dosage was. That was Patricia's job.

"She only has some diarrhea," Patricia said.

"That's your body adjusting to the medications. It'll clear up soon," he assured them.

JoAnn spoke up and asked, "Do any of these medications cause hallucinations?"

Dr. Kennedy's eyebrows went up. Patricia's face had a look of uneasy surprise. Andrea leaned against the exam table in serious contemplation.

"Are you hallucinating?" Dr. Kennedy carefully asked.

"No. No. I was just curious. That's all."

"Some people experience Post Transplant Delirium from the high medicine dose and might see things or people who aren't there. It's rare and over time it goes away. If you have any trouble, call Andrea immediately and let her know, otherwise, we'll see you in two days. Get your labs that morning." Dr. Kennedy stood up, shook hands, said goodbye, and left the room.

Andrea stayed for a while longer to look over her bruised abdomen and her scar that resembled the Mercedes Benz logo; an upward cut in the center of her chest, then a downward slice on each side held together with metal staples. "Everything is healing nicely and it's draining well," Andrea said.

JoAnn had a thin tube in her abdomen that drained any fluid from her surgery. Patricia emptied it twice a day and cleaned around the site. It would remain there until day 21.

They thanked Andrea, asked about the time for their next appointment, then left the liver department and walked silently down the hallways where they passed patients, doctors, nurses, and visitors.

Some patients were in wheelchairs, pushing walkers, or moving slowly and a few had bandages on their arms from the morning labs. Some looked completely healthy. Doctors could be in suits, white jackets or blue surgery clothing. Nurses and clinical staff wore color-coded uniforms depending on their departments. Visitors could be cheerful or dismal, depending on who they were visiting and what the projected outcome of their loved ones was.

Mayo Clinic was always a hustle and bustle of activity. It was clean, modern and emitted an overall feeling of positive health and renewal. The place beamed with hope!

They went outside to the crowded parking lot to their rental car. JoAnn was tired and closed her eyes as Patricia drove back to the beach house.

JoAnn was happy to be back to what she considered to be her *'home'*. She settled down on the porch swing while her sister made them lunch. She wasn't sure what lunch would be, but she knew it would be something healthy since her sister took pride in making wholesome natural meals.

The swing went back and forth in a smooth comforting rhythm, like rocking a baby. The soft voice whispered in pace to the swing's movement. *'Change the baby... change the baby...change the baby'*.

JoAnn opened her eyes and the pretty young lady dressed in a flowered sundress, with long blonde hair, blue eyes, and sun freckled nose, leaned over her and smiled sweetly.

* * *

The Alley Cat, Bar & Grill, was tucked away in a side alley in Neptune Beach, Florida. Over the door entry was a black cat cut out in wood with its back arched. Under the menacing cat was the name of the bar in Old English Type painted in gold leaf. The establishment didn't look very inviting; the big front glass window was covered with a black curtain; the wooden sides of the building were weatherbeaten and the stone steps leading to the doorway were crooked. It looked like the kind of place a person went to hide, get drunk, or to forget their problems. Patricia wasn't going to do any of those things, but opened the door and went inside anyway.

The interior was dismal with low lighting. There was a long bar with barstools on one side, tables in the center, and booths against the wall. There was a coin-operated jukebox against the wall between the restrooms; Tom Cats and Missy Cats. A young couple was seated at one of the booths, eating a pizza and engaged in muted conversation. Glasses and a half pitcher of beer were on their table.

The general mood of the bar was one of peaceful seclusion from the outside world. Bill was behind the bar, sorting through papers. He looked up at Patricia, then returned to his task of organizing papers.

She approached boldly and took a seat on the stool across from him. "Hello," she cheerfully said.

He nodded but didn't look up.

"Nice place."

"What would you like to drink?"

"Nothing. I just came to talk."

He looked up. His soft brown eyes locked on hers. "There's nothing to talk about. This is between myself and my son."

"Really? I got the impression you didn't want to rent the beach house to us."

"That's right. I don't have anything against you personally, but I don't want you there. I'd like for you to leave. I can give you the rent money back."

"I don't want the money back. I want to stay. Besides, I paid for two months although I only expect to stay there for one month for my sister's recovery. She needs to be near the Mayo Clinic for her post-liver transplant appointments."

"Look, if you have enough money to pay for two months when you only need it for one month, then you can afford to get a fancy condo or hotel for her. I'm sure it would be more comfortable than a run-down beach house."

"The house isn't so bad and besides that, we like it. It's rustic and homey. Just what we want and it's a short walk to the beach. You should fix it up a bit and rent it out for extra income."

"I don't need extra income."

Patricia looked around the bar as if reminding him that the place was almost empty. She didn't have to say a word.

"It's off-season. Business is slow."

There was a strained silence between them. He looked back down to his papers. "Find someplace else, will you? Stop causing problems."

Patricia smiled. "Sorry. No. We're staying. Nothing you can do. I signed a contract." She stood up and hoisted her tote bag over her shoulder. "I paid for two months and now, that you're being such a pain in the butt, I think I'll stay for two months."

Bill glared at her from over the bar.

"See ya." She walked out of the bar giving him a goodbye wave.

Float like a butterfly, sting like a bee.

--Muhammad Ali

Chapter Five

It was a chilly February day with a light misty rain. JoAnn didn't think it ever rained in Florida. Florida was supposed to be sunny. Beaches were supposed to be bright and warm. That's why she chose to get her transplant at the Mayo Clinic in Jacksonville.

Carl had been frustrated with her because he said there were plenty of good transplant centers in Atlanta and she should go there. They were just as good as Mayo and family could visit. But she decided otherwise.

As a child, her family would rent a cottage on the Jersey shore and she spent summers by the ocean. When she had her own family, they vacationed on Cape Hatteras, North Carolina. She loved being by the ocean and was insistent on going to Florida to enjoy the sunshine. Now there was no sunshine.

She walked slowly through the house. It was a small two-bedroom cluttered with unnecessary furniture. Patricia's bedroom had a window facing the neighbor's fence, a queen-size bed, a big dresser, a nightstand, and a ceiling fan. There was hardly enough room to walk around the bed, which was probably the reason Patricia gave her the smaller room. The smaller room had a single bed, a small dresser, a nightstand, a ceiling fan, and a window view of the backyard. Unlike the other rooms in the house with used furniture, JoAnn's room was newly furnished with modern DIY (do-it-yourself) buildable furniture. All the stuff that had been in the room before must've vanished.

The bathroom was small with a toilet jammed in close to the tub-shower. There was a shower curtain with big butterflies that matched the window curtains and the rug. The medicine cabinet over the small sink had a butterfly sticker in the corner.

The living room was open and contained big overstuffed furniture, end tables, standing lamps, an oval coffee table, a colorful rug, and two seascape photos on one wall. There was a huge window covered with blue vertical blinds to give a view of the porch, front yard, and road. The living room blended into the kitchen space.

The kitchen area had a small round table with four chairs. The remainder of the room had appliances and countertop space. On one of the counters was a white binder with *'Liver Transplant'* on the front. JoAnn called it her *'Book of Courage'*. Inside the binder were lined pages where Patricia kept a record of JoAnn's weight, blood pressure and when medications were administered. Cellcept, Prednisone, Bactrum, and Prograf were just a few needed to keep her new liver healthy.

To the left was a door to the garage and straight ahead, a door to the backyard. JoAnn went to the back door, opened it, and stepped outside. The gentle ocean breeze was damp and chilly. She wrapped her arms over her chest for warmth.

The yard was blocked by the side of the garage to the left, a wooden fence in the back, and another wooden fence to the right. Everyone kept their beach rentals private which was important when in such close proximity. JoAnn had no doubt the properties on the other side of the fence were much nicer and better maintained than the backyard of their beach house. This yard was a tangle of weeds and unattended dried dead plantings in sandy soil. Perhaps, long ago, when dinosaurs roamed the earth, it was green and trimmed, but on this day, it was a dismal wasteland. The only nice thing, on the small porch, where she stood, was a shell windchime with jingle bells, and ceramic butterflies. As the breeze moved the windchime, the sound was light and cheerful.

JoAnn listened to the sound and thought she heard whispering between the motion of the butterflies and shells. *'Change the baby... change the baby... change the baby'*.

She turned slowly, carefully, and went into the house, closing the door gently behind her. She knew she was losing her mind. She believed it was the medication, perhaps the anti-rejection medication. She wasn't going to ask Dr. Kennedy about hearing voices and she wasn't going to mention it to her sister. They'd think she was crazy, and perhaps she was, but she had no intention of being shipped off to a mental hospital.

She plopped down on one of the soft chairs in the living room and sunk into its comfort. She placed her hands over her abdomen, feeling the rise of the stitches from her surgery. Her thoughts drifted to her donor. Who gave her the gift of life? A man, a woman, old, young, mother, father? How did her donor die? Car crash, heart attack, bike accident, drug overdose?

There were certain criteria for pairing donors to recipients; medical emergency, compatibility, and location. Important factors were the blood type, tissue, organ size, and wait time on the transplant list. Other considerations were the distance from the donor to the transplant hospital, donor and recipient ages, and their medical history. A person who received the gift of life needed to be healthy enough to survive the surgery. An organ was a gift not to be wasted.

JoAnn was grateful a match for her was quickly found. It felt like it was a miracle in so many ways. In a few months when she felt better, she'd write a thank you letter to her donor family and hopefully she'd get an answer to her question, who gifted me a liver?

JoAnn was lost in thought in the living room.

Patricia entered the house carrying a bag of groceries and another bag from a clothing store. "Hey, you're awake! How are you feeling?" She dropped everything on the kitchen table. As usual, she was a flutter of energy and activity.

"Good."

"I bought you some new pants and a top. Something loose that won't bother your stitches. You can try them on later."

"Okay, thanks."

Patricia dug into the food bag. "I'm thinking of vegetable soup and a banana for lunch. How's that sound?"

"Perfect."

"And look!" Patricia pulled out a rotisserie chicken sealed in a plastic container and held it up for JoAnn to see. "For dinner, I got a chicken just like mom used to make!"

Patricia and JoAnn laughed together. Their mother only made processed meals when they were growing up and it was a shared childhood memory.

Patricia prepared lunch. JoAnn sat at the table and watched her wash and chop up fresh vegetables.

Patricia said, "I have good news. I went to The Alley Cat and talked with Bill, Rick's father, the landlord, and he said we're welcome to stay here for two months instead of one. Isn't that nice? Would you like to stay for two months?"

"I would, but don't you have something else you need to do?"

"Me? I'm retired. I have nothing of importance to do."

"I thought you were going to a yoga retreat in Massachusetts or something like that."

"I can cancel. I'm sure I can find a fun yoga place around here."

JoAnn was silent. She wasn't into yoga and doubted she'd ever be able to twist her body up in any contorted weird position to attain enlightenment. JoAnn just wanted to have enough energy to get on with her life, doing simple things and enjoying being alive. She had always enjoyed decorating the house she'd shared with Carl and now she had plans for her condo. It gave her joy to rearrange furniture, change wall paint, select new rugs, hang curtains, and sometimes just simply add a bouquet of flowers to a pretty vase.

She looked around the dingy kitchen and envisioned how she'd decorate it up; paint the discolored cabinets white, a new stove, perhaps a better refrigerator, and a new kitchen table with modern chairs. The place definitely needed an upgrade, but what could she get done in two months with just having a liver transplant? And, why did she want to do anything at all?

"Soups up!" Patricia cheerfully announced.

A butterfly reminds us that there
is always beauty at the end of pain.

Chapter Six

JoAnn sat on the exam table. Dr. Kennedy listened to her heart and told her to take deep breaths as he listened with his stethoscope on her chest and back, and then he placed his fingers on her wrist to check her pulse. He asked her to lie down and he looked over her surgical scar, gently pressed around, then used his stethoscope to listen to any unusual gurgling. All quiet. He told her to sit up, then he went to his computer and studied the morning's blood work. The transplant coordinator, Andrea, stood by with a pleased smile. She knew JoAnn's healing was going along perfectly.

"Numbers look good. How do you feel?"

"I feel great." She wasn't going to mention the voices in her head.

"We'll keep you on this medication for a while. Let me know if you get any side effects."

"Okay."

"Are you walking around?"

Patricia said, "We're staying at a beach house and we hope to walk on the beach this afternoon."

"That's a great idea." Dr. Kennedy stood up, shook hands, and smiled. "See you in two days." He left the room.

Andrea said, "Make sure you get enough rest. Don't overdo things. Don't eat raw seafood. Wash vegetables and no grapefruit or clementine oranges. Keep the drain site clean and draining. And wear a mask out in public. There are germs out there and you don't want to get sick. You have a compromised immune system."

Patricia and JoAnn nodded together. After Andrea looked over the reports in the *'Book of Courage'* and was happy with what she read, she sent them on their way.

JoAnn linked her arm with Patricia's arm as they crossed the parking lot. "Do you think it's okay if we went out to lunch?"

"Sure. Andrea didn't say we couldn't do lunch, just no sushi. Where would you like to go?"

"I'd like to go to The Alley Cat."

"That's not much of a lunch place; it's just a bar and grill." Patricia wasn't overly interested in another encounter with the grumpy disagreeable Bill.

"It's past one o'clock so I'm sure we can get something simple."

"Okay, yeah, sure, why not?" Patricia answered, but she could think of a zillion reasons why *NOT* to go to The Alley Cat.

* * *

Patricia held JoAnn's hand and walked her across the bar to one of the booths. She was happy her sister wore a germ mask because there were people in the bar. A foursome at another booth, a single businessman at the bar counter, an elderly couple at one of the tables and, of course, Bill going from behind the bar to the back kitchen to serve for the *'rush hour'*. They sat down, looked over the menu that was conveniently on the table, and waited.

Bill, dressed in blue jeans and a t-shirt, saw them and seemed to cringe, but walked over. He welcomed them with a friendly smile. "What can I get you?"

JoAnn was quick to say, "I'd like the grilled cheese and fries."

He didn't write anything down. The menu was simple and he knew it by heart. He looked at Patricia and forced a smile. "What about you?"

"You don't have a very healthy menu, but what's the soup of the day?"

"Clam Chowder."

"Is that New England or Manhattan Clam Chowder?"

"New England."

"Okay, I'll have a small bowl of that please."

"Anything to drink?"

JoAnn gave a short laugh, "I'll take a Shirley Temple. I don't drink alcohol anymore out of respect for my liver donor."

He flashed a genuine smile that made him look handsome. "Excellent reason not to drink."

Patricia said, "I'll have a glass of Sauvignon Blanc."

"I'll be right back with your drinks." He turned and left.

"This place is so cute," JoAnn whispered. "It looks like a place where poets and authors would hang out. You know, get on stage and recite their works of art. So much fun. I love this place."

"It looks like a dive bar to me. I'd expect to see a drunk saunter in off the street and beg us for money."

"Why are you so negative?"

"Not negative, realistic."

They sat in silence. JoAnn fiddled with the condiments on the table. Patricia checked her cell phone messages. Patricia put her phone away when Bill returned with their drinks.

JoAnn said to Bill, "I think it's so nice of you to let us rent the beach house for two months instead of just one."

Bill looked directly at Patricia. His eyes flashed with annoyance. Her eyes sparkled with mischief. "No problem. You're welcome," he lied.

"I really like the beach house. It could use some fixing up to make it more comfortable. Would you mind if I did a little decorating?" JoAnn asked.

"Uh, you don't need to do that. You can just leave it as is."

"It might help to entice more people to rent for the summer."

"I don't usually rent it out. You're a special reason."

"Well, thank you."

It was Rick who brought out their food. He placed the plates down and smiled at JoAnn. "How are you feeling?"

"I feel good. Dr. Kennedy says I'm right on track. I was just thanking your father for letting us stay for two months. It will give me plenty of time for my recovery."

Rick didn't bother to look at his father. He knew he was in big trouble. "Glad you're doing well. Enjoy your meal." He turned quickly and returned to the back kitchen area.

"Yes. Enjoy your meal," Bill said with a sincere smile. It wasn't JoAnn's fault. Patricia and Rick were the ones to blame. And, the thought of JoAnn decorating the beach house had his stomach in a knot. He didn't want people in the house and he didn't want anything to be disturbed. He'd locked up the house 23 years ago and wanted it to stay closed forever. He returned to the safety of the bar and washed glasses that didn't need to be washed. From time to time, he looked up to see Patricia and JoAnn talking and enjoying their drinks and food which aggravated him. He wanted them to leave.

The foursome in the booth left, and the businessman got a phone call and stepped outside. The elderly couple left, then Bill went to collect Patricia and JoAnn's plates. "Was the food okay?"

"Wonderful," JoAnn said. "My sister has been making me eat wholesome natural foods, but I really wanted something simple and basic."

Patricia reminded her, "You need to watch what you eat. You have a compromised immune system."

"Oh geez, if you tell me that one more time I'll die."

Patricia was horrified. "No dying allowed!"

Bill smiled a genuine smile. "They do a lot of transplants at Mayo. I'm sure you'll be fine."

"Can we have our bill now?" Patricia asked.

"No charge. This is on the house."

"Really?" Patricia asked, surprised that Bill actually sounded sincere and friendly.

"Yeah. It's our Mayo transplant discount."

JoAnn laughed. "Well, thank you. I'll take that!"

Patricia and JoAnn walked arm-in-arm out of the bar. Once outside in the alley, JoAnn said, "I think Bill is handsome and so nice, what do you think?"

"Yeah. Nice guy."

"I think he has a thing for you."

"A what?"

"He likes you. I can tell. He kept looking at you from the bar."

Patricia hid a smile as she thought, *'Yeah, looking at me because he wants to strangle me.'*

Today I choose gratitude

Chapter Seven

Patricia found a good yoga place and was gone. There'd been a series of warm sunny days and they'd been able to walk on the beach. JoAnn had stood in the sunshine with her feet in the water. It felt good to feel good. She enjoyed hearing the waves and watching the seagulls. She'd picked up a few interesting seashells and Patricia found a shark's tooth. It was good to walk in the sun and they promised to do it every day to help with JoAnn's healing. It brightened their moods as they shared a sisterly bond.

As children, Patricia was the smart one, the chosen one, the one who was the go-getter and geared for success. She had achieved wealth and professional accomplishments. JoAnn was the good quiet child who did what she was told and stayed in the shadows, waiting to be saved and taken care of. She did what she thought she was expected to do; be a good wife and mother. But now, with her generous donor's gift of life did she have a second chance to be someone else? What could she do to honor her donor? What would her donor expect from her? Did she owe something to her donor? Was she supposed to start going to church? Save the world's poor? Start a program for disadvantaged youths? What was expected of her now?

Currently, she liked living in the little beach house, except for the hallucinations and voices, it was a good place to be. She felt peaceful and, as odd as it was, she felt needed, because she needed to *'change the baby'*, whatever that meant.

And so, she stood in the kitchen in front of the closed door that opened to the garage and wondered what was behind it. The garage was under the apartment occupied by Rick who was working at The Alley Cat for the afternoon. The garage was the only part of the house she'd not ventured into, because, what could possibly be behind that door that would be interesting? Most definitely, junk.

She reached out for the doorknob and it didn't turn. It was locked. Where was the key? Did she need a key? It was an old doorknob, and the lock was a skeleton key size, so she went to a kitchen drawer, found a thin butter knife, inserted it in the lock, fiddled around, and unlocked it. She slowly opened the door and peered inside. It was dark, but not so dark that she couldn't make out the shape of a car and a whole bunch of clutter. She reached around the corner for the light switch and, when flipped up, the light blasted into a brilliant view of garage junk.

The car, parked in the center, was a 1965 light baby blue Mustang convertible. She didn't know much about cars, but she did know a vintage Mustang when she saw one. The top was down and the white interior and the entire car were covered in dust. It hadn't been moved or driven in many years. Surrounding the car, but not touching it was old furniture that looked like it had been recently moved into place. She suspected Rick had moved items from the beach house into the garage when getting ready to rent.

There was enough room for her to walk around the car and, she took a leisurely stroll around, daring to place her hand on the car's cold metal hood to feel its history.

Who had driven the car? Why was it hidden away in the garage? Was Bill saving it to sell when the vintage price was right? It seemed like a waste of a wonderfully fun vehicle. She would've loved to cruise up and down A-1-A with her hair blowing in the wind being young free and full of adventure. It was an exciting fantasy except in reality; the car was a manual shift and who could drive one of those things? She doubted the engine would even start.

She stepped away from the car and returned to the door. She turned to give the Mustang a final look and that's when she saw the faint image of the young woman seated behind the steering wheel. She had her hands on the wheel with her head down on her hands. She slowly raised her head, and with tears streaming down her cheeks, said, '*Please change the baby*'.

* * *

Rick parked his black Wrangler Jeep in the driveway and got out. He was finished helping his father with the lunch crowd and was taking a break to do some surfing before he went back to the bar. It was a sunny day and the waves would be good. He saw JoAnn standing on the porch as if she'd been waiting for him. He gave a friendly wave and she waved a greeting that he couldn't ignore. He went over to ask how she was feeling.

"I feel good. Patricia and I have been walking the beach every day. It's nice that this place is on the beach block and an easy walk."

"Yeah. Perfect location."

"You know Rick, I was just wondering why your father doesn't rent this place out and doesn't seem to want to fix it up."

"Yeah. I'm trying to get him to see the financial value of it."

JoAnn carefully asked, "Who lived here before you rented it to us?"

"I only know about my mom and dad living here. Mom died after I was born and after that, Dad closed it up and walked away. Painful memories I guess."

"What was your mother like?"

"I dunno. My grandmother told me very little about my mom. Dad never mentions her. I do know she was a bit of a flower-child hippie. When my grandfather died, my dad inherited money, so they bought this house and the building for The Alley Cat. It was their dream to open the bar for artists to recite poems, read from their writings or sing, or whatever."

"Do you know what your mother looked like?"

"Not really. Dad hid away any photos, but I found one of her in the backyard when she was pregnant with me. She was standing in the garden wearing a flowered sundress and a floppy sun hat. She was smiling with her hands over her belly. Long blonde hair and a freckled nose is about all I know."

"Is that her car in the garage?"

Rick smiled a sheepish grin. "So, you got into the garage."

"It was easy."

"Yeah, I know. When I was a kid, and we lived in the apartment over the bar, I would sneak over here and sit in that car. My grandmother said it was *'Rebecca's baby'*. Silly as it was, to sit in it, made me feel close to my mom."

"I'm sorry."

"Nothing to be sorry about. That's how things play out sometimes. You have something in common with my mother."

"I do?"

"She was an organ donor."

"How do you know?"

"I found a packet with envelopes in it from UNOS, United Network of Organ Sharing. I don't know what the letters say. Dad never opened them." Rick was solemn for a moment, then shrugged his shoulders. "I believe my mom would be happy knowing her death helped others to live."

"Yes. Organ donation is a wonderful gift." She thought about her second chance at life.

Rick noticed her faraway gaze. "You, okay?"

"Fine. I'm fine. Are you surfing today?"

"Yes. I'm going to change into my wetsuit and get my board."

"Can I come?"

He laughed. "Surfing?"

"No silly. Just to walk to the beach with you and watch."

"Cool. That would be nice."

JoAnn watched him walk up the staircase to his apartment over the garage. She now knew who the ghost woman in the beach house was, Rebecca the spirit who wanted so desperately to *'change the baby'*. Perhaps the baby blue Mustang convertible in the garage needed an oil change. She chuckled, but then became serious. What did Rebecca want? Why was she reaching out to her?

Rick took her arm and carried his board under his other arm as they walked to the beach. He let go of her hand and sprinted for the ocean. With a few swift strokes, he was out to his happy place, the surf.

She stood on the shore and watched as he caught an occasional wave. Maybe he was the best surfer in the world, or maybe he was the worst one. It didn't matter because, as she watched, inside her there was a warmth for the young man, a feeling of a mother's love for a son. It was another bond between herself and Rebecca.

Just when the caterpillar thought her life was over, she began to fly.

Chapter Eight

JoAnn stood in the bathroom and dried herself off with a fluffy yellow towel. She looked at herself in the full-length mirror on the back of the door. What the hell had happened to her once slender body? She had bruises on her arms from the IVs and bruises around her abdomen where the staples held her insides closed. She'd be marked for life, but it was a loving scar. She stood in the small bathroom and touched each staple.

"I thank you for my gift. I love you. I love your family. I'm grateful for my life. I'm sorry for what happened to end your life. I touch this one with gratitude. I am blessed," she said and continued with thankfulness until each metal piece was touched.

She wondered why her life had changed so drastically and how her life had miraculously been saved. It all seemed like an unexpected dream that started slowly, then spun out of control. She only remembered some of it.

In the beginning, her gastroenterologist said she needed to select a transplant center because eventually she'd need a new liver, and, although she lived in Atlanta, she selected the Mayo Clinic in Jacksonville Florida. She did some research on their transplant statistics, doctors, and their concept of *'patient centered care'* which sounded good. And she wanted to have a reason to go to the beach when she needed to go to appointments.

She was on medication for five years and struggled with the side effects. Prednisone made her hair thin and gave her a puffy moon face. Her skin was itchy and dry. Her bones and muscles hurt. Her physical ailments were beginning to be a struggle.

Four months ago, Dr. Kennedy noticed a change in her numbers. The most important being the ALT (Alanine Transaminase) which are the enzymes in the liver that convert proteins to energy for liver cells. And the AST (Aspartate Transaminase) which is an enzyme that helps the body breakdown amino acids. There were other numbers out of whack: Bilirubin, Albumin, Protein, Creatine and INR (International Normalized Ratio) which indicated her blood's ability to properly clot. He said she needed to be evaluated for a transplant.

The evaluation process took a week of physical testing to be certain she was strong enough to survive. Receiving a liver was a gift of life that everyone took very seriously. She met with her team: hepatologist, surgeon, coordinator, social worker, nutritionist, financial counselor, and pharmacist. She had blood tests (24 tubes), chest x-ray, CAT scan, Echocardiogram, Ultrasound, and Psychological and cognitive evaluations. When finished her MELD score (Model for End-Stage Liver Disease) was a 9 which was low on a score of 6-40. The higher the score, the closer a person was in need of a liver.

She went back to Atlanta and got her bloodwork taken each week which was sent to the Mayo Clinic for review. Her MELD score slowly rose to 19, but that was in the middle and she wasn't in immediate need. She called Patricia, Carl, and her children to keep them aware of her health. They were concerned, but when they pressed for details, she said very little.

In truth, soon she could barely get out of bed and walk short distances. She'd do small tasks only to return to bed for a nap, then wake up to move around to do more tasks, and then go to bed early. She ignored the signs of liver damage. She covered up her yellowing skin with makeup. She was experiencing *'brain fog'* and couldn't do easy math or make decisions. She had tremors, nausea, and pain in the upper right belly. Her liver wasn't working properly and the toxins in her brain were impairing her daily life. Each day was a depressing struggle to live, but she continued on, pretending she was fine and not in immediate need of a new liver.

One of her preparatory tasks was to put together a *'to-go'* bag because, according to her liver team when a suitable liver became available, she needed to be ready *'to-go'*. Her situation was becoming ominous. She sat on the floor in her closet, selecting loose-fitting clothing, her favorite slippers, a cell phone charger, a toothbrush, hair clips, and a paperback book. She took things out, put things back in, and couldn't decide anything because her brain wasn't working properly and her hands were shaking and then, JoAnn burst into tears and cried. Her liver disease became a harsh reality.

But JoAnn wouldn't give up. She'd fight to stay alive. She was determined to see Beth graduate from college and to welcome her new grandchild into the world. There was still plenty of living she wanted to do. This wasn't the time to die.

On one particular day, she woke up feeling unusually tired, and put eyedrops in because her eyes looked a bit yellow, but decided to continue with her daily plans. She had a meeting with the interior decorator to discuss patio furniture for her condo, and then she went to the outpatient clinic for her weekly blood draw. She could hardly wait to take a nap, but after her bloodwork on her way home, the nurse at the lab called her with the bad news. Her bilirubin, creatine, and INR were through the roof! Her MELD score was 38 and she needed to go to the emergency room immediately!

JoAnn didn't believe her, but drove home to pick up her *'to-go'* bag, then called a taxi to take her to the emergency room and explained the situation to the medical staff. Someone must've called the Mayo Clinic because she received a call about having a liver available for her. It was a miracle match! Most people waited months or years for a donor. She was shocked!

She couldn't think straight, but she needed to get to Florida as soon as possible. She called her sister twice (because being in a toxic *'brain fog'* she forgot she'd already called her) and then everything went into a complete blur. She remembered being wheeled into an ambulance and her mind was drifting in and out. There was no pain. There was no panic. In fact, there was a feeling of peaceful acceptance.

And then there were a bunch of people in the room, washing her up, asking questions, and putting IVs in her arm. It was organized Mayo Clinic precision like a NASCAR pitstop. Out of nowhere, there was Patricia, asking her how she was feeling. She said she felt fine.

Patricia eventually told her, "We're waiting for your donor liver to arrive at the airport."

When her new liver arrived, the surgeon told her it was a good strong healthy match. She told them thank you.

She was moved to a gurney, then wheeled down hallways into the operating room. The room was brightly lit from above with huge concave lights. Everything was clean, sanitized, and white as white could be. The surgical team was smiling and lifted her from the gurney to the operating table. They were still smiling when they strapped down her arms, legs, and head. IVs were inserted in her arms and the anesthesiologist leaned over, smiled, and said something about going to sleep. And that was the end of the world JoAnn had lived in.

Now she stood in the small bathroom, looking at her bruised stitched-up body. She drained the abdominal fluid bag, wiped around the opening, covered it up, and sighed.

Her mind was clear as she thought about her donor and donor family. She loved them with all her heart and soul, but she wondered how she'd been the fortunate one to receive their loved one's liver. She'd done nothing of great value in her life. She didn't volunteer at food banks or walk in fundraisers for childhood cancer. She wasn't a college professor, doctor, political advocate, or social worker. She spent her days picking out furniture and paint samples, decorating and redecorating her condo. Her children were adults and didn't need her. She didn't have a spouse to share her life with. She had lived a simple existence for herself.

Was it divine intervention that gave her a second chance at life? Were the planets of the solar system in alignment on that day? Did her horoscope predict it? Perhaps her donor chose her to receive the gift of life. But why? Why? Why was she chosen to get a second chance at life? Now what?

JoAnn sighed and pulled on her loose-fitting sweatpants. She positioned the pants to hang below her treasured scar. She pulled on her baggy sweatshirt, brushed her teeth, combed her hair, and felt a bit better… perhaps more deserving.

She took a final glance around the bathroom and said aloud to no one except herself, "This place needs some new wallpaper. Yes. I think I'll pick out some samples and start some redecorating. And, that bathtub has got to go! Nobody uses bathtubs anymore. A nice walk-in with new fixtures will really look nice." This thought, although not much, gave her life purpose, which was what she needed now.

Chapter Nine

Patricia knew she looked *'hot'*. She was dressed in her yoga pants and yoga top and wore a light jacket and sneakers. She'd never had children; her belly was as flat as a pancake and as tight as a drum and her breasts were perky as a teenager. For a fifty-five-year-old, she was toned muscle, and in perfect health. She ate healthy, exercised, and read all the labels on her food. She wore her hair in an attractive style and occasionally had the grey dyed out. She had few wrinkles, but they were signs of her wisdom.

She stepped lightly into The Alley Cat and was glad to see Bill alone behind the bar. She dragged a barstool out, sat down, plopped her tote bag on the counter, and smiled. "Hello."

"Hello."

"I just finished with my yoga class and I thought I'd stop in for a drink."

"What'll you have?"

"I don't suppose you have any coconut water back there."

"I can make you a pina colada if you'd like."

"Maybe a glass of Zinfandel."

"Yeah, that goes good with yoga." He smiled and she smiled back. He reached for a wine bottle and a glass, filled the glass, and placed it on the counter.

She took a small sip of wine. "My sister really likes the beach house. She's into decorating and this morning she was looking over wallpaper for the bathroom."

"I'd prefer she leave it as is."

She took another sip and studied Bill. She remembered Rick telling her that his parents had lived in the beach house until his mom died, then Bill locked it up and walked away. She had no doubt the house brought back painful memories. She wanted to ask how his wife had died but decided against it.

He moved away from the bar and she sat alone, drinking a few more sips, then she stood up, carried her glass, and went to the jukebox. She looked over the tunes and noticed one of them had a strip of black tape covering the choice. She turned her head to study Bill moving around behind the counter and sadly realized the tape probably covered a favorite song of his and his wife. She looked back at the jukebox to make a different selection, then gasped.

He looked at her.

"Oh my God! This is coin-operated! Nobody has coins anymore! How can it even work?"

He left the bar, walked to her and stood close. "It's free now. Just punch your buttons."

"Well, that's nice." She smiled and felt an odd sense of excitement blended with quiet comfort. He was so close she could reach out to kiss him. She could smell his cologne, or was it an imported beer scent? Belgian Ale? She stood still, finger on the letter 'A'. He stood still, looking into her face. They could kiss and they both moved slightly forward as if to make it happen. She closed her eyes but felt nothing on her mouth. He had stepped away.

She was disappointed. She pressed the letter 'A', then the number '17'. The record moved out of the slot, dropped into position and Kenny Rogers sang *'Just Dropped In To See What Condition My Condition Was In'*. The music choices were as old as the jukebox --very old.

Patricia went back to her barstool and thought her jukebox selection was perfect. He must've thought so also because he shook his head and smiled. They'd established a truce.

* * *

The dream came slowly and it was wonderful! JoAnn was sitting in the passenger seat of Rebecca's convertible. Rebecca was driving, grinning from ear-to-ear and tapping her fingers on the steering wheel to the loud music; The Beach Boys singing *'Help me Rhonda'* blasted from the radio. Rebecca and JoAnn's hair was blowing in the wind as they sped down A-1-A towards Jacksonville Beach with the top down. It was a perfect sunny beach day!

JoAnn looked to her right side and, although they were zooming quickly along, the buildings were passing by slowly, as if trapped in time. They passed Mellow Mushroom, The Dairy Queen, Taco Bell, and First SunTrust Bank. JoAnn was filled with happiness, joy, and excitement. Life was absolutely wonderful and she turned to look at Rebecca to tell her how great she felt.

Rebecca wasn't smiling. She looked mad, no - - more than mad, she was furious! She took her hands off the wheel, grabbed JoAnn by the shoulders, and yelled, *'Change the damn baby'*!

The Mustang swerved to the right, bounced up and over the curb, flipped sideways, then landed on it's side, skidded down the sidewalk with metal scaping the cement, and crashed head-on into a palm tree.

They whispered to her,
'you can't withstand the storm'.
She whispered back,
'I am the storm.'

Chapter Ten

JoAnn jumped out of bed, smacked her knee into the nightstand, and crashed against the wall. She was shaking and frightened.

Patricia ran into the room. "What's wrong? What happened? You fall out of bed?"

"No. No."

"Did you pull your stitches out?"

"No. No. I'm fine."

"You don't look fine. You're shaking. Come on, let's take your blood pressure." Patricia took her hand and led her into the living room, where she put her in a soft chair then went to get the blood pressure gauge. She checked her out.

JoAnn's blood pressure was high, but not bad. "You scared me." Patricia, who was not easily frightened, confessed.

"Yeah sorry. I had a nightmare. Rebecca tried to kill me."

"Who? What? I don't know any Rebecca."

"Rebecca is Bill's dead wife. She was driving her Mustang with me as her passenger and she crashed it *on purpose*. She tried to kill me."

Patricia sat silent, processing the bizarre information.

"She's haunting this house. It's her house and that Mustang in the garage is her car. She's mad at me for touching it."

"It was just a dream."

JoAnn nodded. "Yes. Just a dream."

"Do you often see this…uh…Rebecca person?"

"Yes, but she's a ghost."

"Well, I've never seen her."

"That's because you don't believe in ghosts."

"I didn't know you did."

"Lots you don't know about me. Why should you know everything?"

"I would've liked to have known there was a ghost haunting this house." Patricia stated firmly, then added, "We can find a new place if you want."

JoAnn stood up. She was calm. "I want to stay here. I have to *change the baby*."

Patricia watched her sister slowly walk down the hallway to her bedroom and close the door.

She was worried but didn't know who to call for help. It was a little after twelve o'clock at night. Perhaps Bill was still at The Alley Cat.

Bill answered the phone.

"Hi Bill, this is Patricia. I'm sorry to bother you. Are you busy?"

"No. Just closed up. Wutzup? Something wrong? You got a plumbing leak?"

"No. It's my sister. She's acting weird."

"Weird how?"

"I think she's hallucinating."

"With her transplant, you should be calling her coordinator, not me."

"She says she's been seeing your wife Rebecca's ghost."

Silence.

"JoAnn had a dream that Rebecca was driving a Mustang and crashed it so JoAnn would be killed."

Silence.

"JoAnn said she touched Rebecca's car in the garage and now Rebecca's mad. Is there a Mustang in the garage?"

"I told Rick not to let anyone in the garage. It should be locked."

"So, there's some truth to this isn't there?"

"Look, why don't you just gather up your stuff and go to a hotel? You shouldn't be in the beach house. And you shouldn't be nosing around where you don't belong. I'll give you your money back."

"I don't want my money back. I want answers. I want to know why my sister is hallucinating and seeing a ghost. Can you come over?"

"No."

"Please."

"No. Good night."

"Please."

Silence.

"Just come talk with JoAnn. Please."

"Not now. Maybe in the morning."

"Thank you."

"Yeah, right." Bill clicked off the phone.

Patricia sat in the silent darkness, looking around through the moonlight shadows, wondering if Rebecca's ghost was watching her. She shivered.

Courage does not always roar,
Sometimes it's the quiet voice at
the end of the day saying,
I will try again tomorrow

--Radmacher

Chapter Eleven

Bill stood in the driveway. He felt sick. The beach house was one giant threatening sorrowful place to Bill and he didn't want to go inside. He was nervous and broke out into a cold sweat. His heart beat rapidly and he couldn't breathe.

The door opened. Patricia greeted him with a warm 'hello'.

"Good morning," he somberly replied.

"Come inside."

He cautiously and slowly walked up the steps and into the house of anguish.

The interior wasn't as Bill remembered. Rick had rearranged and changed out some of the furnishings. He'd replaced the living room wall paintings with modern colorful framed photography to make it more *'rentable'*.

Patricia was cheerful. "Rick did a nice job fixing it up. Take a look around," she said and waited for him to take a tour.

He didn't want to take a tour. He wanted out of the house! But he wandered down the hall to the larger bedroom, the one he'd shared with his wife. There was a new bedspread and mattress, but his memories of making love, laughing, and pillow talks with his wife came back as a painful reminder of what he'd lost. He stepped quickly away and glanced into the bathroom. Yes, perhaps JoAnn was right and it needed new wallpaper, maybe an upgrade to a walk-in shower.

He stopped in front of what had been the baby's room. Gone were the Winnie-the-Pooh stickers, the soft animal mobile, the baby crib, the flowery curtains, and the changing table. Everything was replaced with furniture from a box that Rick had put together. It was ascetically pleasing, clean, fresh and it was full of JoAnn's things instead of baby stuff.

He went into the kitchen where JoAnn sat at the table and Patricia leaned against the counter. There was a new microwave and coffeemaker, but the new sparkling items couldn't erase the memory of Rebecca lying on the floor.

23 years ago, he found her curled up in the fetal position beside the kitchen table where her cup of morning tea remained untouched. She must've stood up, then crumpled to the floor, passed out, and went to sleep forever. He wasn't with her. She died alone. He had to catch his breath as, once again, the vision and guilt flooded into his mind.

JoAnn's voice broke his miserable thoughts. "Good morning, Bill."

"Hi."

"Patricia didn't tell me you were coming over. Is something wrong? Would you like a cup of coffee?"

"No thank you," he answered and looked to Patricia for her to explain things to her sister.

Patricia spoke slowly and deliberately, "I invited Bill over because…"

There was a tap at the front door, then Rick hurried inside and said to his father, "I saw you drive up. Can't you just let it go and let them stay?"

Bill answered, "I have no problem with that."

"Then why are you here?"

"Patricia invited me over."

Everyone looked at Patricia, who looked like a deer caught in the headlights, stunned. "I uh, I'm concerned about JoAnn and what she told me last night. JoAnn you want to tell them about your dream?"

"Not really. They'll think I'm nuts. It was only a dream."

"You said it was a very vivid dream, very real."

JoAnn was silent for a moment, gathering her thoughts, then explained, "I guess it makes sense now that I think about it. I went into the garage to look around and I touched Rebecca's car. I don't think she liked that very much and so she appeared in my dream. It was cool in the beginning, we were speeding around in her car listening to beach tunes, then she grabbed me by the shoulders, yelled at me to *change the baby*, turned the wheel and we crashed into a palm tree. I think she wants to kill me."

Bill shook his head. "That's absurd. Rebecca wouldn't even kill a spider in the house. She'd take it outside and put it in the garden."

JoAnn smiled, "Yeah maybe, but what if the spider was on her car, *Rebecca's baby*?"

There was silence as everyone wondered about spiders, cars, and dreams.

Patricia said, "Tell them more. Tell them about Rebecca's ghost."

"You can believe me or not, but I've seen Rebecca's ghost in the house. She comes and goes, but mostly she likes to sit on the porch swing. Sometimes she tells me to *change the baby*. I thought she was friendly until now."

"If this is real, and you're not hallucinating, then maybe we should get to the bottom of this," Patricia said and reached for the doorknob to open the garage which had remained unlocked since JoAnn had previously ventured inside. She opened the door, turned on the light and 23 years of musty dusty smell immersed around them.

One by one, they went through the doorway and into the cluttered garage. Rick had piled it up with furniture, but he'd be careful not to put anything against his mother's 1965 baby blue Mustang convertible.

JoAnn warned, "Don't touch her car."

They didn't touch the car but stared at it in awe. Bill remembered how much his wife loved driving the car, polishing it, pampering it with oil changes and new tires. It made him smile. He looked around and saw parts of the baby's crib with Winnie-the-Pooh, Piglet, and Eeyore stickers. Rick had taken the baby furniture apart and stored it in the garage. The crib was behind the baby changing table. The plastic pad on the changing table was yellowed and dusty; the drawers closed shut.

JoAnn slowly said, "That's a baby changing table. Rebecca keeps asking me to *change the baby*. I wonder...." She stepped forward and gently opened the top drawer, and that's where she found the journal on top of the dried unused baby wipes. She picked it up carefully, knowing and appreciating its value; a baby book for her son from his deceased mother. She turned and handed the book to Rick.

Rick held the book, blinking back tears, staring at the white cover with butterflies and the words; *Baby's First Year*. He was unsure if he wanted to open it, and so he passed it to his father. "I don't think I'm ready for this Dad."

Bill held the journal in silence. His heart pounded and he was uncertain if he wanted to even hold it. Rebecca had started the journal when she found out they were pregnant and it was a loving record of Rick's arrival. One page was marked with a thin lavender silk ribbon. He fingered the ribbon, but like his son, he wasn't sure if he was ready to read Rebecca's words.

Rick turned, said nothing, and left the garage and went up the stairs to his apartment. Bill waited for a moment, then he quietly left the garage, passed quickly through the house, got in his car, and then drove away.

Patricia and JoAnn turned off the light, left the garage and closed the door. Patricia got the bagels out to heat in the toaster oven for breakfast. JoAnn sat at the table to finish her coffee. She smiled and said, "Well that went very well, don't you think?"

A butterfly lights beside us like a sunbeam
And for a brief moment its
glory and beauty belong in our world.
But then it flies again
And though we wish it could have stayed...
We feel lucky to have seen it.

Chapter Twelve

Bill walked into The Alley Cat, grabbed a bottle of Jack Daniels off the bar, and headed up the stairs to the apartment. He carried the journal tucked under his arm.

He spent the remainder of the day walking past the journal on the coffee table, taking sips of whiskey to get his courage up. He knew he had to open the journal, but he also knew it was going to be heart-wrenching to relive Rebecca's death.

He finally sat on the couch and opened the journal to the last entry, the one marked by the soft lavender silk ribbon. It was the morning she died.

* * *

It had been a restless night for the three of them. Rick, only five weeks old, needed to be fed every two or four hours and Rebecca was exhausted. Bill had gotten up, changed the baby, and brought the baby to their bed for her to nurse. When she finished, he burped the baby, and then put him down to sleep. Bill had suggested they start bottle feeding so she could rest because she always looked pale and tired, but she'd hear none of that!

And so, as he stood in the kitchen that morning, she sat at the table dipping her tea bag into her tea cup and rubbing her temple. She had another horrible headache.

"You look tired," he said.

"I'm fine."

"I think I'll stay home with you today."

"Don't be ridiculous, you have the plumber coming."

"I can cancel. It's not that important."

"I think getting the plumbing done at The Alley Cat is important. We need bathrooms."

The Alley Cat was in the beginning stages of making their dream a reality. It was a lot of work to renovate the space and open a bar. He thought the bar, and their newborn, were causing unnecessary stress for her. "Do you still have a headache?"

"Yeah, but the tea will help."

"Take something for it will you?"

"I don't want to take anything because I'm breastfeeding. I'll be fine. I'm a bit nauseous."

"I'll make you some toast."

She shook her head, smiled, and said, "Just go to the bar and meet with the plumber."

"No. I'm staying here. I'm worried, okay. How's the pain under your ribs?"

Rebecca stared at her coffee cup and blinked her eyes as if trying to focus on what was in front of her. "What?"

"Do you have any pain?"

She laughed, "Just you. Now will you go!"

He stood silent, worried, and unsure what to do. "I think I should take you to the ER."

"I'm fine. Would you stop worrying so much."

"Okay, look, I'll come home at noon okay."

"You don't have to do that."

"No, but I want to."

"Okay."

He leaned over and kissed her cheek. She smiled and waved him away like a troublesome gnat.

At 11:45 his world crashed to pieces. He knew something was wrong as soon as he stepped into the house and saw Rebecca lying on the kitchen floor. He kneeled beside her, shook her to wake up, then tried to check for a pulse. He was so nervous and upset, that if there was a pulse to be felt he couldn't feel anything. He dialed 911 and, in a gasping frightened voice asked for immediate help and explained the situation. "What? I don't know if she's breathing. How old is she? I dunno… uh 23… can you get here *NOW*? She just had a baby five weeks ago. I don't know. I don't know. I don't know. Why are you asking me all these questions? I gave you our address. Just get here!"

EMS (Emergency Medical Services) arrived with lights flashing in their white-yellow truck. The police showed up with their flashing blue lights and the fire department whirled in with sirens. Rick, who'd been asleep, woke up and added to the noise with his crying.

Bill stood stunned and confused as people moved quickly around him, asking questions, pushing him aside, and telling him to give them her medical and health information. He watched two men pick Rebecca up and put her on the gurney. "Is she alive?" he asked.

"Yes. We got a pulse."

Another man said, "We'll take her to Mayo, is that okay?" The medical technicians exchanged glances as if knowing something was seriously wrong and a transplant center would be a good choice because her medical information indicated she was an organ donor. If she died, her death could save many lives.

Bill answered, "Yes. Yes. Sure. Mayo Clinic is good." He didn't care where they took her as long as she got help.

They wheeled Rebecca outside to the ambulance. Bill hurried behind.

"You want to ride with us?"

"Yes! Yes! Can I?"

The policewoman came out carrying Rick who was crying. "You go ahead. I'll call a social worker to look after the baby. We'll bring him to you at the hospital."

Bill had forgotten about Rick and was thankful someone was thinking more clearly than he. He climbed into the ambulance, they shut the door, and he held Rebecca's hand all the way to the Mayo Clinic. He asked her to stay strong. He told her she'd be fine.

At no time did she move. At no time did she open her eyes. At no time did she squeeze his hand. At no time did he give up hope that she'd sit up, open her eyes, and say something, anything!

Silence.

Your scars are the stars
You won in the Dark Phase of Life

--neha

Chapter Thirteen

Rebecca died of a rare condition, Postpartum Preeclampsia. They missed the warning signs: high blood pressure, headache, upper belly pain, nausea, blurry vision, and, in the end, a seizure. She had lain on the kitchen floor for three hours with no blood flow to her brain and now Rebecca was technically brain dead.

Bill stood by her bedside in the hospital for a week, waiting and watching for any sign of life. She didn't open her eyes or move.

There was no one to notify. Her mother had died when she was fourteen and her father was a free spirit who was last seen sailing in the Caribbean to unknown destinations. He called his mother in California who quickly flew in to help with the baby and to help with possible funeral arrangements. Taking care of Rick kept Bill busy and this made him thankful so he could forget that his world had fallen to pieces.

Rebecca was on life support with a ventilator to keep her alive. On the monitors, there was a flat line where brain activity should've been recorded. Her heart was strong and her breathing was being assisted, but she was lifeless. He sat in the lounge with his mother and the medical team as they explained she'd never recover, but she was an organ donor and her death could save the lives of others. It was what she would've wanted. A decision had to be made sooner than later. He felt helpless.

He was still in denial that she was dead. What if she wasn't *really* dead? What if everyone was wrong? What if she would open her eyes tomorrow, a day after they took her off life support? What then? They could be wrong! Then she'd *really* be dead!

He finally accepted the fact that Rebecca was brain dead. That morning, he signed the consent forms for organ donation and already suitable recipients had been found. He didn't know where her organs were going, but he knew it was what she would've wanted. It was what he would do. The surgical team was waiting for him to say his final goodbye.

He stood by the bed, holding Rick in his arms. He looked at Rebecca. She was pretty with her long blonde hair, sun-freckled nose, and pink lips. She looked so peaceful and so healthy that he hoped she'd smile, open her eyes and give him her cute little laugh. She was still. She was silent.

He didn't tell her he loved her on the morning she died. Of all the days to forget to say a simple, *I love you*, it had to be that morning, that day, the last day. How could he have been so thoughtless? He always said he loved her when they parted, but not on that day.

And although it was too late, he mumbled, "I love you." He was hopeful she heard him.

He placed Rick in her arms and folded her arms around him. A gush of tears fell down his face and he sobbed like he'd never sobbed before. He cried for the years she'd never know. He cried for the future they'd never share. He cried for the missed ballgames, graduations, marriages, and grandchildren she'd never experience. He cried for lost Christmases, and birthdays, cooking burgers on the grill, building sandcastles, and playing in the ocean waves. He didn't know if he cried for her, or for himself, but he cried as Rebecca lay still holding their sleeping baby in her arms for a final time.

He wasn't a religious man, but he reached out to God, begging to die in place of Rebecca, making promises to go to church, read the Bible, and to be a better man if only she would live. There was no bargain to be made and his pleas were lost in the silence of the hospital room.

When he could cry no more and when he was an emotional wreck, he took Rick from Rebecca, gave her a kiss on the forehead, wiped his tears on Rick's baby blanket, turned, and left the room.

The hallway was empty except for his mother, who gave him a sympathetic smile, wrapped a kind arm around his shoulders, led him away, and said, "Rebecca will give others the gift of life. She will be remembered and loved by many."

Bill wasn't in the mood for love and forgiveness. The anger and rage came like a hot iron on his heart. He was angry at Rebecca's Obstetrician for not keeping better watch on her. He thought he might sue the practice just to be mean. He hated the people who disconnected her from life support and blamed them for her possibly dying before her time. He was angry at the plumber he had to meet on the day she died. It was the plumber who made him leave her alone.

He yelled at everyone who came to help him renovate The Alley Cat because they needed to be yelled at. The world was dismal and he hated living in it without Rebecca.

He shouted at his mother for touching or moving Rebecca's things and she finally called him a *'jerk'* and went back to California, leaving him alone with a newborn baby.

He was angry with Rebecca for dying. She should've let him take her to the ER that day. Why was she so stubborn? He should've known something was seriously wrong. Why had he been so stupid? It was his fault. It was her fault. It was the world's fault.

Rick was his only reason to live and he held on to him as a source of hope, but even that wasn't enough and he replaced his baby with booze. Drinking liquor made it all go away and he sank into a dark depression. He was numbed to the world but that was better than feeling the emptiness of not having Rebecca in his life.

The years passed, and as Rick grew from a baby into a boy, Bill realized he needed to let go of the alcohol and focus on being a good father. They played ball and video games together, went on hiking trips, fishing, boating and took an overly expensive week at Disney. But always there was an empty hole where Rebecca should've been there with them.

* * *

That was 23 years ago and in a different lifetime. Now he finally had the courage to confront the past. He slowly picked up the journal and opened it to where it was marked. He read her words in hopes of finding comfort. Rebecca had written in the journal after he'd left to meet the plumber.

Today I woke up tired again and my head won't stop pounding. I know something must be seriously wrong with me. When your father gets home, I'll let him take me to the ER. But I think the tea will help and I can nap with you lying in my arms, so maybe I will feel better. I love you and your father so much that I can't bear the thought of dying and leaving you two alone. I will always be with you.

Bill closed the journal, set it on the table, and stared at it. Of course, she didn't want to die. She didn't want to leave him and Rick, but that's how things happened. After she died, he tried to move on with his life; opening The Alley Cat like they planned, taking care of Rick, and finding small things to busy his mind.

It took him awhile to accept that there would always be a missing piece in his heart, but that was okay because he was comforted knowing the memory of her was forever with him.

Because he'd been overcome by the discovery of the journal, he didn't open The Alley Cat that night, but instead spent the time pondering the past; feeling sorry for himself, and drinking. Now he had to continue with his life. It was time to *'let go'*.

He stood up and went downstairs to the bar. It was dark and empty because it was ten o'clock in the morning and closed. He went into the small storage closet and moved around the condiments.

Behind the box of sugar cubes was Rebecca's ashes in a pretty flowered urn with her birth and death dates elegantly scrolled in gold leaf. Beside the urn was an 8 ½ x 11 manila envelope with UNOS handwritten in faded black ink. Although Rebecca hadn't been with him through the birthdays, vacations, and life's milestones, by the giving of her organs, she had gifted these wonderful life events to six other people.

Under the envelope was a framed photograph of Rebecca standing in the backyard garden smiling with her hands on her pregnant belly. She was surrounded by flowers, sunshine and butterflies, living in joy, happiness and hope. This was Rebecca. This was the gift of life she wanted others to enjoy.

He carried the items to the bar and grabbed a step stool as he passed it. He positioned the step stool to the back of the bar, and moved expensive bottles of liquor to make room for the urn. That's where he placed Rebecca's ashes and photograph -- in a place of honor and love where she could see their vision as a reality.

He stepped down, studied the urn for a moment, then went to the front window. It was closed with dark moody curtains, but now it wouldn't be like that anymore. He opened the curtain and bright sunshine blasted into the once dismal bar. He stood in the sunlight, and was filled with a sense of love and harmony as he embraced only happy memories of his life with Rebecca. She would've been proud that he'd continued with their dream.

Although she was no longer with him, he realized that the giving of her organs gave others their lives. She gave others the joy of living. What better gift could there possibly be?

He called Patricia to invite himself over, then he called Rick and told him to meet him at the beach house.

* * *

JoAnn and Rick sat on the porch swing. Bill and Patricia sat in separate chairs. Bill handed Rick the envelope and asked him to please read the donor recipients' letters out loud; Terry, Sarah, Lori, Steve, Maria, Jim. The letters gave basic information about the organ recipients, no addresses, only information about their lives, their families, their hopes, dreams, aspirations, and their reason for needing an organ. Each letter overflowed with gratitude and thankful words.

When Rick finished reading everyone was joyful and smiling. There was a warm feeling of peaceful closure. Rebecca was put to rest; they *changed the baby* and *changed their lives* as she had changed the lives of so many others with *the giving of life*.

*To receive gifts with grace is a gift to the giver.
You're allowing them to have the experience
of being 'one who gives'.*

Terry

It was a summer when parents went to work in the morning and kids were told to go outside and play, don't get in trouble, and to come home when the sun goes down. And so that's what Terry did. He rode his bike to Frankie's house to meet up with his buddies (aka: The Rider Gang). Their first stop was in the woods at the rope swing over the pond behind McDill's farm.

The five ten-year-old boys were dismayed that the pond looked unusually muddy and funky. Should they try the rope swing over the pond and drop down? Was it safe? Would they get stuck in the mud? The water was lower than usual but maybe it was deep enough.

Terry, who was the lightest kid, was voted to try it out. He willingly volunteered because he wasn't going to *'chicken out'* in front of his friends.

The rope hung on a branch of an old oak tree and beside the tree was a mound of rocks piled up to be the jumping-off point. Terry took off his shirt, socks and shoes, reached for the rope, kicked off the rocks, swung out over the water, let go of the rope, flew free into the air, and then plopped headfirst into a stinky bacteria infested murky pond. He sunk to the bottom, got his hands and feet stuck in the muck, and came up gasping, choking, and looking like *'The Creature from the Black Lagoon'*. At some point, he swallowed some of the dirty water and Terry didn't know it then, but his life was about to change.

The Rider Gang was stunned and then burst out laughing as they dragged Terry to safety. It was decided that swinging over the pond was a bad idea. They'd ride over to McDill's farm stand to get some candy instead. They washed Terry off with a garden hose and he didn't stink so bad anymore.

The next morning Terry woke up with a bad stomach ache but dismissed it because The Rider Gang was going to play baseball at the school field. His position was shortstop and he had to be there. That night he wasn't very hungry and complained to his mother that his entire belly area hurt. She gave him some Pepto Bismol and sent him to bed. This continued for a week until one morning, he had a fever, but ate some cereal which he threw up. The Rider Gang showed up to check on him but found him asleep in bed, so they left him alone. That's where his mother and father found him and that's when they took him to the emergency room with bloody diarrhea, a high fever, confusion, fatigue, and gripping abdominal pain.

The Rider Gang, frightened and distressed, fessed up to Terry's head dive into a contaminated pond. It didn't take long for the doctors to diagnose Hemolytic Uremic Syndrome (HUS). He had swallowed e-coli and the toxin-producing bacteria were destroying his red blood cells and injuring his kidneys. They tried blood transfusions, plasma exchange, and the medicine Soliris, but he was beyond dialysis and in complete kidney failure. He needed a new kidney and was placed in UNOS for immediate need.

As Terry lay in the hospital bed his parents stood by his bedside and The Rider Gang held vigil in the parking lot. He was in and out of consciousness and almost dead. Terry vaguely knew what was going on, but he knew he was in serious trouble. Whenever he opened his eyes, he could see his mother crying or his father's worried face. Through blurry vision he saw concerned doctors and sorrowful nurses. He hated himself for causing so much sadness for so many people. Eventually Terry *pretended* to be asleep so he wouldn't have to see what was going on.

Although his eyes were closed, he could still hear people talking. *'He's so young, this is so sad, he's just a boy and has his whole life ahead of him, will they find a kidney in time?, will he die?, this is such a shame, he's so young, dear God please, please save my son, stay strong, don't give up'.*

The only person Terry opened his eyes for was the Phlebotomy technician who came by at five o'clock in the morning to draw his blood for his labs. The technician would ask how he was feeling, he'd say he felt fine and the technician said he looked good. They were good liars.

One day the technician came in and said, 'don't you worry none. I heard them talking and a nice young lady named Rebecca gifted you a new kidney. You're gonna be just fine. Treat that young lady right ya hear me?'

Terry nodded that he most definitely would take good care of his gift of life.

The doctors came into his room, packed him up and put him in an ambulance for the transplant center two hours away. Everyone was happy and joyous as the hospital staff waved goodbye.

The Rider Gang, on their bikes pedaling like heck, followed the whaling flashing ambulance to the edge of town where they stopped to wait for his return.

Upon arrival at the transplant hospital, Terry was prepped for surgery and waited to see if the kidney was a suitable match, and when it was, he went into surgery. Four hours later he woke up with IVs in his neck and arms and his parents asking him how he felt.

Terry felt great! His new kidney immediately began its job, clearing out his blood and filtering all the bad stuff. He stayed in the hospital for two days, enjoying the desserts and watching TV while lying in bed. When he returned home, The Rider Gang came to see his scar which they viewed with admiration and respect. He was a superman. He was a survivor! Terry knew his donor was named Rebecca, but he wasn't going to tell the gang he had a new *'girl'* kidney. Terry would love Rebecca forever.

Playing it forward, every day

Sarah

Sarah hated the way she looked. Tears pooled in her eyes as she studied herself in the full-length mirror. What had happened to her? At one time she'd been a thin woman with tons of energy, but now she was fatigued, fat, and connected to an oxygen tube in her nose to help her breathe. It happened three years ago after her daughter was born. The decline was slow and her struggles went unnoticed for a year. Soon she couldn't walk very far without being out of breath and getting dizzy. And she started gaining weight.

Her sister gave her diet plans, her mother scolded her for not taking better care of herself, and her doctor told her to get outside and exercise. Her husband began to help more with household chores and her oldest daughter would try to make her laugh because she was always in a sullen mood. She couldn't hold on to her full-time job as a retail manager because of her fatigue, then she went part-time, and then the company politely *'laid her off'*.

They had to live on her husband's income and there was barely enough money to pay the bills, so there were no planned vacations or money to fix up their three-bedroom house. They did have his health coverage which was proving invaluable since she was constantly at the doctor's or the emergency room. 'I can't breathe,' she would say, but nobody listened.

Finally, an observant doctor became suspicious of her many visits to the ER and began a series of tests to determine what was wrong. She had blood tests, a chest x-ray, an echocardiogram, an exercise stress test, a CT scan, an MRI, a lung function test, a sleep study, a lung biopsy, and then a right-heart catheterization which diagnosed her with Pulmonary Arterial Hypertension.

PAH is a progressive disease that affects the precapillary pulmonary vasculature. There is no cure. The cause is unknown. It is a progressive disease and eventually will lead to a double lung transplant, or if untreated, fatal heart failure.

Sarah immediately went on a series of drugs, and oxygen therapy 24/7, but for the next two years, she continued to decline.

Sarah could barely function. She tried to clean the house, but doing any task left her dizzy and exhausted. She attempted to cook a meal, but that proved hazardous with the oxygen tube dangling out of her nose. Her mother helped with the kids while her husband was at work, but her mother didn't believe she was really sick and often told her to *'suck it up'*.

She couldn't drive. She had a huge oxygen concentrator at home, but for outdoor trips, she had a portable oxygen concentrator, which enabled her to go to the stores or to her oldest daughter's softball games. She hated going out because of how people perceived her to be: overweight, slovenly, slow, and lazy. And the diarrhea from the medications was horrible! When going out of the house, she was humbled to wear adult diapers because she never knew when her bowels would let loose and she'd be in an awkward situation.

For a while, she had a rollator (walker with wheels), but even that became difficult and then she was stuck in a wheelchair. She felt like a burden and an embarrassment to her family. Sarah was depressed and hated herself.

She and her husband had discussed getting a lung transplant with the doctors and weighed the risk factors, which were high. Sarah said she didn't want to live the way she was living anymore. She wanted to be there for her husband and her children. She had always wanted to travel west to see the Grand Canyon, Yosemite, Carlsbad Caverns, and stick her toes in the Pacific Ocean at Big Sur. There were things she wanted to do. She wasn't ready to die. She'd take the gamble to live for herself and her loved ones. She was placed on the transplant list and waited for a suitable donor. She was heartbroken to think she was waiting for someone to die, but she desperately prayed for a pair of lungs.

As she cried and looked at herself in the mirror, her husband came and held her in his arms. He attempted to console her with kind words and kisses. 'I love you. We'll get through this. It's not your fault. You're beautiful. Don't worry. They put you on the lung transplant list. Maybe we'll get a call soon'.

Days passed into weeks, that passed into months, and then after a year of waiting the call came. Sarah struggled off the couch to call her husband, who rushed home immediately. She called her mother to come watch the kids. She packed what things she thought she'd need. Her transplant coordinator said they were flying in healthy lungs and it looked like it was *'a go'*. Fingers crossed! They kissed the kids, hopped in the car, and zoomed down the highway.

Sarah was hopeful. Her thoughts weren't on the difficult recovery ahead, but instead on the future of a new life with her family. She'd be able to walk across a parking lot and not gasp for breath, she could wash the kitchen floor without getting dizzy, drive to her children's activities, bake cookies for the school bake sale, make love to her husband, and there were just so many wonderful things she'd be able to do with her second chance at life.

At the transplant center, Sarah was prepped for surgery and met the transplant team who assured her the lungs were a good match. Her husband kissed her and said he'd be waiting for her when she got back to the room.

Ten hours later, Sarah opened her eyes and saw her husband smiling at her. She had a tube down her throat and couldn't talk, but gave him the thumbs up, which made him smile.

She remained in the Intensive Care Unit for two weeks and laughed when she was released and the doctors told her she shouldn't go bicycle riding, jogging, or do aerobic exercises for at least 4 more weeks. Sarah just wanted her life to be how it had been, and now she had a chance to be a mother and a wife again. It was a wonderful gift given to her by a generous donor.

She went into physical therapy, and was soon back to enjoying her daily activities. She felt fine and began planning for a trip to the western states, but there was a heaviness hanging over her joy. She was overcome with guilt and torment.

She believed, that by her constantly asking for a pair of lungs, she asked for someone to die for her to live. She was responsible for her donor's death. She was a horrible selfish person!

When her husband came home, he found her crying in their bedroom and when he asked what was wrong, she sobbed that she was fine. But Sarah wasn't fine at all, she wanted to stay in bed and do nothing. Her feelings of guilt took over her life. She went to her daughter's softball games, but there was no joy to see her play. She would stop reading a book to her youngest daughter, close it, and say she needed to rest. She wouldn't rest. She'd cry - - cry because she was enjoying her children and another person, her generous donor lost the happiness that she was enjoying. She cried for the donor family and the loved one they lost. What were their lives like now without their loved one? It was her fault she was alive and her donor was dead. She felt shame, sadness and guilt.

Sarah and her husband went to the transplant center for her checkup and her husband mentioned to the doctor about her possible depression, mood change, and constant crying.

She denied it all. 'I'm fine,' she lied.

Fortunately, the doctor didn't believe her. He said some people feel the way she was feeling after a transplant. She had *Survivors' Guilt* which was similar to PTSD (Post-Traumatic-Stress-Disorder). He said having a transplant can be a traumatic event causing sleeplessness, anxiety, detachment from living, and mood changes. He immediately made her an appointment with a therapist.

Sarah went to therapy and learned coping skills to overcome her guilt feelings. She learned to focus on breathing, do morning journaling, and to stay grounded with the day's activities. She joined transplant groups at the hospital and as time went by, she was able to enjoy the wonders of her life and she graciously accepted the giving of life granted to her.

It took two years before she had the courage to write to her donor family. To pursue her love for traveling, she added Arches National Park to her *'places to visit list'*. She was going to find the biggest arch in the park and place a bouquet of flowers beneath it in thankful gratitude to her donor. Her healthy lungs were a bridge from death to life.

Lori

Lori sat in Dr. Medford's office and couldn't stop crying. She had used up half the tissues in the tissue box and held a bundle of tear-soaked tissues in her hands. Heart failure? How'd that happen? A heart transplant? They can't be serious, can they? Oh, but they most certainly were serious!

Her mother was also tearful, but her father, the army sergeant was stone-faced. Doctor Medford's face looked so gloom-and-doom that he frightened Lori.

She never thought all the testing would result in such a disastrous outcome. There had been blood tests, a chest x-ray, an electrocardiogram, an ejection fraction, a stress test, a CT scan, a heart MRI, a coronary angiogram, and a myocardial biopsy. The diagnosis was clear and final; she had Rheumatic Heart Disease caused by her having undetected rheumatic fever as a child when they lived in Korea.

She was now 21 and, other than one doctor mentioning a heart murmur, she'd been healthy with no heart issues. She was a dance major enrolled in her second year at the College of Charleston. Dancing was her love, her life, and now it was being taken away. Her world was shattered. Her dreams vanished into the next handful of tear-soaked tissues.

She didn't catch any of the signs that her heart had a stiffness that made it no longer functional. She thought the hard exercising for her dance classes made breathing difficult. And, there was the weight gain which she couldn't explain because she ate very little, and in fact, eating made her nauseous. Her arms and legs began to swell up and she looked *'puffy'*. Her hands and feet were constantly cold. She was fatigued to the point of always just wanting to lay down to rest.

But there was no rest. There were classes to attend with her full course load. There was practice, practice, practice. There was study, study, study. There was party, party, party. It went on and on and on until the Friday night she became confused and lightheaded to the point that her roommate took her to the campus health center. It ruined their Friday night plans to attend a Frat Party and it was the possible beginning of the end of Lori's dancing career.

She wanted to get her degree in dance studies, and maybe do a few dance gigs on stage, perhaps dance behind a rock star, but her ultimate dream was to open a dance studio so she could share her joy and love of dance with others. She was even including some education and business classes in her busy college schedule.

It had been too much. She pushed too hard. She had big dreams. She had her bright future planned out -- until now.

Her father asked Doctor Medford the important questions: how long will the wait be for a heart donor, what's the cost, are there medications to help while she waits, how long is the recovery time, who will do the surgery, can she recover at home, can she continue with college?

Everything went unanswered. No guarantees. It was *'waiting without answers'*. Just like the military, hurry up and wait. And so, Lori did that.

She dropped out of college and went home with her parents at Fort Bragg. As she waited for a new heart, she stayed in her room and moped around in her black leotards feeling sorry for herself. She closed the curtains and only came out of her room to barely eat enough to support a bird. She lost weight. She didn't go out with her friends and in fact, refused to see or call them. She blamed her father for them being stationed in Korea where, perhaps the medical care wasn't good. She blamed the army for sending him there. She blamed her mother for not seeing what was wrong and getting her help when she was a baby. She blamed her brother for her getting a bad heart and his heart was fine!

It was the world's fault she had a bad heart and she was mad as hell!

She became so angry, mean, nasty and depressed that her parents sent her to a therapist.

Doctor Ellington asked her what her fear was.

Lori confessed: This isn't my fault. I didn't ask for any of this. And now I'm dying. I'm going to die. I've done horrible things. I'm going to go to hell. I'm a mean person. I told Brenda she looked like a baby hippopotamus in that silly pink tutu. I stole Vivian's boyfriend in high school, not because I liked him, but because I knew I could do it. My older brother snuck out of the house one night to be with his girlfriend and I locked him out, so he got caught and was grounded for two weeks. I step on worms. Worms are stupid. They don't have the courage to be snakes or anything cool, they just squirm around without brains. And my heart transplant surgery will be a failure, it's karma. I'm going to get bad karma. The universe is working against me. If they give me a new heart, it won't fit or it will bleed all over the place and I'll die a long painful death. My old heart will explode before I can get a new one. I won't be able to go back to school. I won't be able to dance ever again. If I can't dance, I might as well be dead.

Doctor Ellington told her to imagine she was standing in front of a gentle stream in a peaceful forest. She told Lori to pretend to pick up a leaf, place it in the water, and watch it float away saying *'I forgive myself'*. Pick up another leaf, put it in the water, and watch it float away saying *'I'm letting go'*. And another leaf *'I live in this day'*. And continue with putting a leaf in the stream to watch it float away, *'I give up my worry about tomorrow, I am here today, I am thankful'*.

In time Lori came to understand the lesson, learning to live for each day. She felt herself growing, changing, and accepting the wonders of her daily life. She found pleasure in grocery shopping with her mother, eating popcorn, and watching TV with her father. She called Vivian to say she was sorry for stealing her boyfriend in high school and they both agreed he was a jerk anyway. They renewed their friendship. When her brother came home from bootcamp she confessed that she told on him the night he snuck out and he laughed because he didn't remember that at all. She continued to listen to dance music and, on the days when she felt good, she practiced dancing. Her dancing gave her purpose, a hope, a dream that still might become true.

After seven months of waiting, on a bright sunny day, they got the call that a compatible heart donor had been found. Her mother, being an army wife, had everything packed and ready to go. Her father drove them to the transplant center and she was prepared for surgery. Everything moved quickly and with precision. Doctors, surgeons, interns, anesthesiologists, and nurses came and went.

The surgeon told her how the procedure would be done.

She would receive a general anesthetic before the operation, then put on a heart-lung machine to keep oxygen-rich blood flowing through her body. The surgeon would make an incision in her chest, separate her breast bone, open her rib cage, remove her old heart, sew the new donor heart in place, and attach the major blood vessels. Her new heart would begin beating when the blood flow was restored.

Lori lay down in the operating room, looked up at the lights, and envisioned that wonderful stream in the woods where she placed down a single leaf to watch it float away. She closed her eyes and drifted peacefully to sleep, accepting the outcome, whatever it may be. In her mind she placed a leaf in the stream and said, *'I give it up to the universe'.*

Six hours later Lori woke up. She was attached to a ventilator; there were IVs in her arms and she had tubes in her chest to drain fluids off her heart and lungs. She stayed in Intensive Care for a few days, then was moved to a hospital bed and eventually went home with instructions to come back every month for check-ups.

Lori returned to college for the next semester. She didn't sign up for a heavy course load but decided to take it easy and enjoy her new life. She apologized to Brenda for calling her a baby hippopotamus and she stopped stepping on worms. She still didn't like worms, but she'd let them continue with their life journeys in hopes that eventually, they'd reincarnate into something with a backbone or an exoskeleton.

And odd as it was, in the past, Lori usually wore black leotards and moody dark clothes, but now she chose to wear flowery wispy dance outfits and lowcut shirts to show off her surgery scar -- her *gift of life*. Now her very favorite thing to do was to dance barefoot on the beach wearing colorful sundresses.

If nothing ever changed,
there would be no butterflies

Steve

Steve didn't feel quite right and went to his primary care physician. He complained he was losing weight, tired, and felt pain in his upper stomach and back. He was told he was under stress from getting a new job promotion, buying a big house with a big mortgage, two car payments, and a wife with a baby girl on the way. It was how life was, stressful. He was told to do yoga, meditate, and learn breathing techniques to calm down.

Steve wasn't into yoga, and didn't have time to meditate, but he tried breathing exercises that didn't work so he went to another doctor. He complained he wasn't hungry, had pain under his ribs that flowed to his back, his skin was itchy and his bowl movements produced light-colored poop that floated at the top of the toilet bowl. The doctor told him his body was misaligned and cracked his back, which felt wonderful at the time, but didn't help. The third doctor did some blood tests, gave him opioids for his back pain, and sent him away.

His wife, Janet, thought he was mimicking her pregnancy discomforts and believed he was a hypochondriac. She was tired of him telling her he was going to die, to which she told him, if he died, he should have a life insurance policy. He agreed and took out a million-dollar life insurance policy.

Steve didn't understand why his perfect life had suddenly gone off the tracks. He was an architect in a big firm and had worked hard to achieve financial success. He had planned out his life as perfectly as a high-rise elegant hotel; college, marriage, career, big house, two new cars, 2.5 kids, members of the country club, and fun vacations. He was always feeling sick and that wasn't part of the plan.

He went to a fourth doctor. Doctor Patel spoke with an accent that was so heavy Steve could hardly understand him, but the good doctor rolled his office chair over to him, held his hands, looked into his eyes, and told him he'd solve his problem. That was the first time anyone took him seriously and that was the beginning of Steve's journey.

Doctor Patel did a series of testing that included a CT scan, an MRI scan, a PET scan (position emission tomography), an ultrasound, a biopsy, blood tests, and genetic testing. After everything was done, he called Steve and asked him to come to his office and bring his wife with him. It sounded serious and it was. Pancreatic Cancer. It was the *'BIG C'*. It was a death sentence. His wife burst into tears. Steve was stunned to silence. Doctor Patel showed them the images and pointed out the huge cancer mass in the middle of his pancreas. A pancreas was needed to produce digestive enzymes and regulate blood sugar. Steve's pancreas looked horrible, but the doctor had an attack plan.

First, Steve would go on the pancreas transplant list, but usually, a pancreas was transplanted with a kidney because most receivers had diabetes that required both organs. Because Steve only needed a pancreas, the wait could be longer and during that time he'd be on chemotherapy to keep the cancer from spreading to other organs, which would be a very bad thing.

The treatment schedule would involve multiple injections over a period of three weeks, followed by a rest, then start again. He would experience fatigue, nausea, diarrhea, hair loss, appetite changes, and maybe neuropathy and skin redness.

Steve and Janet's journey began the following Monday. Steve told his boss what was going on and received support from the company to continue working when able. Everyone was hopeful he'd make it through the chemotherapy and quickly get a new pancreas.

With his job secure and knowing he and Janet had saved enough money that they could pay bills for six months, he felt hopeful. As time progressed, the chemotherapy was difficult and he was often sick and tired, which caused him to miss work, but he continued on.

He was in the middle of a conference meeting when he received a call that he was to come to the transplant center because a pancreas had been found. He joyfully announced the news and everyone gave him high-five's as he left the building. Janet met him at home and they rushed to the hospital. He was in his hospital gown and waiting for surgery when he got the bad news that the pancreas wasn't a good match.

The ride home was mostly filled with Janet's comforting reassuring words, but Steve felt devastated. He spent the next two days in bed, depressed.

As the months went on, Janet was feeling the pressure of tending to Steve, keeping the house in order, working as an office manager for an electrical supply company, and her pregnancy. She was exhausted, but there was no one to help them. He could barely do the yard work or trim bushes and things around the house began to fall apart. Their family wasn't nearby to help and they carried the burden of Steve's illness alone.

Because of his absence, the company put him on FMLA (Family Medical Leave Act) which gave him pay for 12 weeks at 70%. The bills began to pile up. There was no one to give them financial help because their families were financially worse off than they were. Janet sold one of the cars to remove a car payment, but that meant she was taking him places and her job performance was becoming an issue. She feared for her job, which would be devastating! They'd lose everything within one month.

Steve and Janet were spiraling into financial ruin. Their savings and the money set aside for their baby's college fund was gone. They only had a few investments available to take out money. Steve was getting worse, not better. It was then that a second call came in for his pancreas transplant and they rushed to the hospital only to be turned away because the surgeon didn't like the way the pancreas *'looked'*. They drove home in silence with Janet blinking back tears. Steve went to bed, depressed, and slept for three days.

As time went by, fewer friends and colleagues called or visited them to check on Steve's prognosis. It was as if people were afraid to hear how he was doing, fearing for the worse, or perhaps they got busy with their own lives and he was forgotten.

One night he had a dream and shared it with Janet. In his dream, he was Jimmy Stewart in *'It's a Wonderful Life'* and sitting in the evil Mister Potter's office holding his life insurance policy. Mister Potter said, *'It looks like you're more valuable dead than alive'*.

When Janet got to work, she called her mother for support. Her mother said everyone was busy with their lives and couldn't help, except Aunt Nancy in Connecticut. She'd help.

Aunt Nancy was 78 years old and flew down like a tornado of positive energy. She immediately began to get things organized. She mowed the lawn, trimmed the bushes, cleaned the gutters, and power-washed the driveway. She drove Janet to work and took Steve to his appointments or to work on the days he felt good. She went to the animal shelter and came home with a '*comfort puppy*' for Steve. It was his responsibility to train, feed, and walk the puppy to give him a sense of purpose.

She helped Janet prepare the baby's room, vacuumed the house, cooked dinner, did the laundry, and did everything that she thought needed to be done - - which was a lot.

Aunt Nancy, through no fault of her own, had buried two husbands and she knew what most people didn't understand. She recognized '*caretaker burn-out*'. Janet was impatient, not eating enough, overacting to simple problems, and she was pale, fatigued and an emotional wreck.

Janet cried on Aunt Nancy's shoulder. 'I can't do this anymore. I'm not strong enough. Each day he gets worse and I'm helpless to save him. I don't want to watch my husband die'.

Aunt Nancy sent Janet off for a massage and pedicure, gave her money to go to an afternoon movie matinée. She gave her a bag of bread-heels and told her to walk in the park and feed the ducks at the pond. Janet said people weren't supposed to feed ducks bread, to which Aunt Nancy said she'd never met a duck that didn't like bread. Janet walked in the park, but didn't feed the ducks. Sometimes a girl had to make her own decisions.

Aunt Nancy could squeeze a buffalo nickel until it farted. She was good with money and finding hidden financial deals. She went with Steve to the transplant social worker to see what was available for help, then sat down with his company's human resources to find support. She downsized their bills by decreasing car and home insurance, got a better phone plan, sold unneeded items at a garage sale, went to the free food pantry, and researched every possible assistant program. She cancelled their fancy club membership and signed Steve up for a book club. She recycled bottles and cans for extra cash, knitted baby bonnets to sell at craft fairs, and for all her hard efforts Steve and Janet had their heads above water and they now believed they'd be able to ride out Steve's pancreatic cancer. Aunt Nancy reminded them; that it was temporary and soon they'd be back on track. They were thankful for her help.

Steve and Janet slowly walked in their neighborhood on the sidewalk with the new puppy on a leash. They shared a heartfelt talk. They realized that all they'd been striving for; the big house, fancy cars, and job promotions wasn't what life was about. They had each other, and a healthy baby girl on the way which was all they needed for a wonderful life. They returned home, sat down, and evaluated their priorities. After Steve's transplant, they'd sell the house (before it was foreclosed on) and buy something smaller. He didn't want to return to his stressful career and they figured, if they stuck to a tight budget, he could be a stay-at-home-Dad. A calm peaceful acceptance surrounded them. It was a wake-up call to change their lives and strange as it was, this in itself was *'a gift'*.

When the third call came for a pancreas transplant Aunt Nancy drove quickly to the hospital with lights flashing and the horn blasting for everyone to get out of her way. When they arrived, the donor organ was a perfect healthy match! All things were *'go, go, go'*!

In ICU Steve woke up with Janet holding his hand. Aunt Nancy was busy in the hallway telling the nurses how to do their jobs. Janet asked him how he felt and he said he felt great. She told him one of the transplant nurses said the donor was a young woman named Rebecca. 'Do you think Rebecca would be a good name for our baby girl?' she asked.

'I think Rebecca is a beautiful name.'

Trust the wait
Embrace the uncertainty
Enjoy the beauty of becoming.
When nothing is certain, anything is possible

--Hale

Maria

Maria was a second-generation Hispanic. Her mother and father came to the United States of America from Puerto Rico seeking a better life for themselves and their children. They worked hard to catch the American dream and bought a house in Miami. They raised their four children, of which Maria was the second born. Maria married Carlos, moved into a house around the block from her parents, and had three boys (ages 4, 7, and 12). She lived a full happy life surrounded by her aunts, uncles, siblings, cousins, and the Puerto Rican community.

Carlos worked as an auto mechanic and Maria was a first-grade teacher. To get her teaching job she had to undergo a complete physical. This was when the doctor told her she had the potential to develop NASH. He explained it was Non-alcoholic Steatohepatitis or in layman's terms: Fatty Liver Disease. She needed to change her diet, exercise, lose weight, and take prescribed medications to keep her cholesterol, triglycerides, and blood pressure at healthy levels.

Maria started out doing well, but as time went on it was difficult not to eat all those delicious Puerto Rican foods: mofongo, lechon asado, arroz con gandules, and pasteles. She was a busy person with her teaching job, her kid's activities, planning vacations, helping her parents, and participating in her community's festivals and events.

Her home was the destination place for every kid in the neighborhood and there was always a full house of people for Maria to love and take care of. She loved all children as if they were her own. She did for others before herself and she enjoyed every minute of it! Going to the pharmacy to get her medications was put on the back burner behind her family's needs and as the years progressed, so did her fatty liver disease.

There were signs she ignored. Her liver was taking in more fat and calories than it could process. She was always tired with unexplained weakness throughout her body. Her judgment wasn't as good as before, she was often confused, forgetful, and couldn't concentrate. She would look at one of her students and forget their name, or write down misinformation about a class lesson plan. She'd forget food recipes that she'd made her entire life. Walking and doing easy housework became exhausting!

She had finished reading a book to her first-grade class and told them it was recess time. They raced outside and she raced to the bathroom where she spit blood into the toilet. She didn't feel well, but thought the blood in her mouth could've come from her teeth. She would need to make a dentist appointment. Her day continued and she went home to prepare a huge meal for Carlos, her three boys, the two girls from across the street, and her cousin who showed up unexpectedly to complain about her rat-bastard husband.

Maria watched them eat, but she ate nothing. She wasn't hungry. She was tired and, after she cleaned up the kitchen, she sat down beside Carlos to watch TV. He placed his arm over her shoulder, brought her close, and kissed her on the lips, then his eyes got really big and he asked if she was ok. It was at that time that Maria projectile vomited blood all over him, her, the coffee table, couch, rug, and pillows. He jumped up in surprise!

Maria didn't remember much after that except Carlos calling 911. She remembered the EMT's showing up and her boys crying in the hallway. Someone told her to *'hold on, stay with us'*. People and voices faded in and out as if in a dream. There was no pain. She was simply bleeding to death. Despite the sirens and flashing lights, for Maria it was a pleasant ride to the hospital.

Eventually, she was able to understand what had happened. She'd had a dangerous life-threating esophageal varices bleed and they needed to immediately take her into the operating room to band and cauterize the ruptured veins in her neck. Bleeding varices happened because there was a blockage in her liver that caused smaller blood vessels, that aren't designed to carry large volumes of blood, attempting to go around the obstruction. The smaller blood vessels had burst under the pressure. After surgery, she woke up with a sore throat, a room full of worried doctors, and Carlos looking like he was scared to death. The diagnosis was stage 4 cirrhosis caused by the non-alcoholic steatohepatitis she'd been ignoring for four years. She needed a liver transplant.

She stayed in the hospital for a week as they evaluated her for a transplant. She was put on medication and sent home to wait with a MELD (Model for End-stage Liver Disease) score of 20. (6 being low-40 being high).

Carlos was worried. Her family, friends, and neighbors in a five-block radius were worried. They stopped by to see how she was feeling. They helped with the boys, cleaned her house, made meals, and picked up her medications. Each week Carlos took her for her bloodwork and as the weeks passed, she wasn't getting better, only worse. She could no longer go to her teaching job.

She kneeled in front of the Virgin Mary statue in their dining room and prayed. She attempted to say the rosery, but couldn't remember the proper order. Maria began to cry and this was where Carlos found her.

She tearfully moaned, 'Why has this happened to me? What have I done to deserve this? God has forsaken me. Why am I being punished? I ask for forgiveness. I ask for my sickness to go away, but each morning I wake up feeling worse. Why have I fallen out of God's grace? What do I have to do to be forgiven for my sins? Why am I being punished?'

Carlos didn't have an answer, but he held her and cried with her. They cried and prayed until Maria suddenly stopped crying. It was as if she was abruptly hit on the head with the answer to her prayers.

Overcome with pure joy, she said, 'This is a test of my faith. I believe in God and his will *will* be done. I will not forsake my belief in God. God will send me an angel to help guide me. I have my faith. I have my faith and that will be enough'.

She went to her weekly blood test with renewed courage, faith, and hope. One day she asked Carlos to take her to the school so she could speak with the children in her first-grade class. She explained to them that she had a sick liver, but she was going to be fine. Some of the children looked tearful and she told them not to worry because an angel was going to bring her a new healthy liver.

It was a slow journey for Maria. She had abdominal swelling known as ascites which gave her a big fat belly. She couldn't walk five feet without running out of breath. She had confused thinking, anxiety, and sleepiness because of the Hepatic Encephalopathy (toxicity in her brain).

The doctors feared she'd slip into a coma before a donor could be found so she was placed in the hospital to wait, or to die. When Carlos sat by her bed, holding her hand, and tearfully said, 'Don't leave me Maria. I can't live without you', she didn't have the strength to reach out to console him, but she had faith -- faith that an angel would save her.

She felt hands around her, lifting her up, putting her down, lights blazing in her face and she knew her angel had arrived!

Maria opened her eyes. She blinked a few times to get her world in focus. Carlos was smiling at her, telling her they found her a liver donor match, the surgery was a success, and she was going to live!

She was on a fast road to recovery and was like a new healthy person. They had her walking the hallways on the second day and she was released from the hospital in four days. She returned home with doctor's orders to get weekly bloodwork done, not to lift anything weighing more than 10 pounds, and to be careful of her belly stitches. In time they removed the abdominal drain and Maria was back to her routine of helping others. As her strength returned, she relished in her second chance to enjoy life.

Maria was scheduled to return to teaching her first-grade class that morning. She stopped by the hospital for her weekly bloodwork and was surprised when the lab nurse looked into her face and shook her head. The nurse said her eyes looked *'yellow'* and asked if she was foggy-headed and fatigued. Maria had been so busy and excited about returning to her job that she figured those symptoms were a result of her pushing herself too hard.

The lab nurse called the transplant center to tell them what was happening, and Carlos came to pick her up to bring her to the hospital.

As they rode in the car, Maria prayed, *'Hail Mary full of grace; The Lord is with thee. Blessed art thou amongst women, and blessed is the fruit of thy womb, Jesus. Holy Mary, Mother of God, pray for us sinners now and at the hour of our death'*. She said the prayer over and over and Carlos prayed with her.

When they arrived, she was immediately placed in a room for *'observation'* and *'testing'*. After a short time, it was determined that her liver was being rejected because her body thought her new organ was a foreign object and her immune system was attacking it. It was a nightmare! It was the worst thing that could possibly happen after a transplant - - *REJECTION*!

Maria had her faith and knew an angel was looking over her and she'd be fine. They adjusted her anti-rejection medication and within a few days, she was sent home with her liver healthy again.

Maria kneeled in front of the Virgin Mary statue and told God that now she'd be more mindful of her diet and her health. She would take care of her new liver. Every night she prayed for God to watch over her donor family in what she knew must be an emotional time of grief and sadness. She felt a loving bond with her donor and donor family, now joined in faith.

Her return to the classroom was only delayed one week. She was excited and happy to be back, but what really surprised her happened when she stepped into her classroom full of smiling children and saw every wall, desk, and cabinet in the room had a hand drawing of a liver from the children. Someone must've shown them what a liver looked like because the pictures resembled smiling happy livers. Some livers had legs and arms, some had hair on liver heads and a few had silver wings and gold halos.

Maria cried happy joyful tears. Not only had her angel come, but she had many angels in her life.

Butterflies are God's proof that
we can have a second chance at life.

Jim

As the story was told, Henry and Yolanda Jones acquired the land in 1865 as part of Special Field Order No. 15 proclamation by General William Tecumseh Sherman that gave freed slaves 40 acres and a mule. Henry and Yolanda selected 40 acres of rich Georgia bottom-land as their tiny piece of paradise, but they were so poor they had to eat the mule and pull the plow themselves (so the story was told). As time went by, they grew enough peanuts to buy a horse to use and as time moved on, they built a small house and had seven children who helped with the farming so they could grow more crops to sell, to make more money, and to buy more land.

There was a time when people thought black people would be best suited to learn a trade or skill and so it was Henry's son William who went to Agricultural College and learned all there was to know about fertilizing, crop rotation, soil compounds, animal husbandry, and getting fresh produce to market. William took the small farm and started expanding it into a huge enterprise. He sent his son, Jacob to Howard University in Washington DC to become a doctor.

The farmhouse was now a huge 12-room, 8-bedroom house with 4 generations living happily on over 1,500 acres of prime growing land. They grew peanuts, yams, cabbages, sweet corn, cucumbers, watermelon, peppers, tomatoes, blueberries, and pecans. They said they'd never grow cotton.

Jim's wife, Patty was a business genius and ran the farm like she was CEO of a big corporation. All employees (mostly family) had fat 401K's, health coverage, a dental plan, and received 5 weeks paid vacation. The farm had tractors, harvesters, plows, seeders, spreaders, irrigation sprayers, mowers, and livestock trailers. The Jones family was the richest family in the county.

Jim had inherited the farm when his father decided to retire, but not only did he inherit the Jones farm, he also inherited his mother's diabetes which killed her when she was only 70. His 86-year-old father told him he got *'the sugar'* (diabetes) from her side of the family. Jim didn't care where it came from, but he was tired of watching his diet, checking blood sugar levels, and having to get dialysis three times a week at the hospital for his failing kidneys.

One kidney was shriveled up like a raisin and the other one was barely functioning. He was stage 5 ESRD (End-Stage Renal Disease) and had maybe 2 years to live. He'd been on dialysis for 3 years and was experiencing low blood pressure, weight gain, and muscle cramps. He was on the kidney transplant list, but since he wasn't *'almost dead'*, but only *'close to being dead'*, he was a low priority.

Jim didn't want to die like this, waiting for a kidney. He would prefer to die while performing some heroic deed, fighting for his country, or at least having a tractor fall on top of him killing him instantly. It wasn't to be so.

Everybody knew Jim Jones and his huge family. Jim was only 60 and tried to help his sons run the farm, but they put him *'out to pasture'*, letting him only do small chores. Everyone on the farm had a job for the daily operations. His granddaughter, 3-year-old Emily would wake him up at 6 am to collect eggs in the hen house. They'd carry an empty basket and fill it up so that it was so heavy Little Emily could hardly carry it, but she wouldn't let PopPop take it from her. Her little face would turn bright red from the strain, but she carried all the eggs because PopPop was sick and she needed to help.

When they returned to the kitchen Patty and the assortment of daughter-in-laws, daughters and granddaughters, and grandsons would prepare a big breakfast. Jim would go upstairs to help his father shave, shower, and dress, then bring him downstairs in time to ring the bell on the front porch to bring everyone in to eat. Everyone would eat in the large dining room, then return to their farm jobs. The older boys drove the younger kids and themselves to school. Jim and Little Emily busied themselves in the vegetable garden, fishing in the pond, or feeding the farm animals. And then they'd take a nap after lunch.

On dialysis days, Patty drove him to the hospital with Little Emily in the backseat. As he sat in his dialysis chair Patty would knit and Little Emily would read a picture book to him, but she couldn't really read so she'd make up stories from the pictures. Sometimes they'd stop for ice cream on the way home.

He was usually tired after that, and not very hungry, but when dinner was ready, he sat at the table with his huge family sharing conversations about the day's events.

It was Jim's job to say the dinner prayer. *'Dear Lord, we thank you for the food we are about to receive. We thank you for this day's labors and the gifts of a good harvest. If a kidney is granted to me by your grace, give us grateful hearts for the donor and donor family. Blessed be to God. Amen'.*

After dinner he'd sit in his favorite loveseat with Patty, holding hands as they watched *Wheel of Fortune* and *Jeopardy*. The rest of the family usually sat in the living room with them to watch TV and every piece of seating furniture was occupied, sometimes with the younger ones on somebody's lap, or laying on the floor. At this time Jim and Patty knew they were blessed to be surrounded by their loving family.

Jim lived in a small town full of friends, people he knew, and people he didn't necessarily want to know. His community knew he didn't need money to help him, but he did need prayers and that's what he got. The people at his church prayed for him to receive the gift of life -- a new kidney. Each Sunday his name was on the top of the prayer list before Helen's foot surgery, Richard's gallstone, funds for a new library, and UGA (University of Georgia) winning their game.

Jim asked God to help him live long enough to see Little Emily graduate from college. Each night his family sent prayers up to God for him to remain alive and healthy so they could have him around for a while longer. There were so many prayers being sent up that God took notice.

The phone call came in the middle of the double jeopardy questions on *Jeopardy*. Jim's family acted quickly with Jim asking if it was for real. Didn't somebody else need a kidney more than he? Maybe he didn't need *that* kidney. Maybe it should go to someone else. He was strong and he might live for at least another few years.

Oh, he was the closest in distance and a good match, so it was real and it was his turn. He kept questioning if he should be the one to receive the gift of life. They reminded him, if he didn't get this kidney, he could die. Little Emily burst into tears, hugged his legs, and said she didn't want PopPop to die. His family ignored his doubts, told him to shut up, and shoved him into the car.

Everyone wanted to go to the hospital and the family piled into five vehicles to get there; the Chevy truck, the Bronco, the Explorer, the van, and Patty's Mercedes. They hurried to the hospital.

To a room full of worried family, the surgeon explained they were going to give him a kidney but leave his other two kidneys in place. The new kidney would help strengthen the old kidneys, and by taking off some of the workload, it would give them a *'kick-start'* to work properly again.

Jim had never heard of such a silly thing, three kidneys? The surgical nurse explained Jim's donor was named Rebecca and now he'd have his two kidneys and one of hers.

As Jim was getting prepared for surgery, his big family hugged him, kissed him, and told him everything was going to be just fine. Little Emily held on to his hand until he was taken down the long hallway to the operating room, then she followed for as long as they'd let her, waving goodbye. 'Bye, Bye, PopPop. I love you.'

Jim's family sat in the lounge -- waiting and praying. A nurse came often to keep them updated on the 3-hour procedure.

Jim's kidney transplant was a success and he woke up in the recovery room with his entire loving family filling every inch of standing and sitting space. He was filled with an overwhelming sense of love, gratitude, and thankfulness for his family and now, for his donor and donor family.

Little Emily sat on his hospital bed and patted his hand to give him comfort. The nurse walked in, speechless to see a room full of people. Little Emily put her hands on her hips, tilted her head, and announced, 'My PopPop has three kinneys and one is named Bekka.'

The miracle of giving is that it ripples.
One small gesture can affect hundreds.

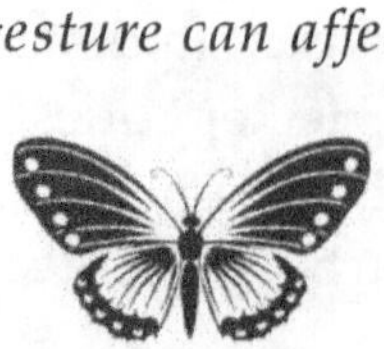

Chapter Fourteen

JoAnn sat on the porch swing and flipped through a book of wallpaper samples. Bill and Rick had given her the *'ok'* to do some decorating to update the beach house. They also agreed to let her rent the place for as long as she liked because, like her, they felt she belonged there. She would go back to her Lake Lanier condo when the weather got too hot. Her healing from her transplant was going well and Dr. Kennedy gave her the *'thumbs up'* to do her own thing. She'd return every 3 months for a checkup, then eventually every 6 months, and then once a year if everything went well.

Patricia also liked living at the beach house and spent a lot of time at The Alley Cat. She'd grown fond of Bill and sometimes after the bar closed, they'd put soft tunes on the jukebox, dance close, and share a few kisses.

Rick read his mother's journal and placed it on his nightstand. He read some of it before going to sleep. It was a loving reminder that she was always with him. He would write letters to the recipients of his mother's gift of life, and although it had been 23 years, he was hopeful they were doing well. He didn't know the whole stories of Terry, Sarah, Lori, Steve, Maria and Jim, but he'd let them know something about his mother.

After Rick had read Rebecca's donor letters JoAnn felt better about receiving her generous gift of life. Many of the recipients were just like her, ordinary people living everyday lives with hopes, dreams, and aspirations that had just been interrupted for one reason or another. They needed a second chance to finish their life journeys and organ donation gave them that opportunity.

She rose from her seat on the swing and decided to take a walk to the beach. It was a nice sunny afternoon and she was strong enough that she could walk long distances without becoming tired. Her new liver was strong and healthy. She was forever thankful to be alive, and although she probably wouldn't do something amazing with her life like run marathons, invent Velcro, or become an astrophysicist, she would relish each day as a blessing and a gift. It was, she knew, what her donor wanted; *for her to live her life in joy*.

When the time was right, she'd write a thank you letter to her donor's family to give them closure.

She walked to the beach, took off her flip-flops, and felt the sand between her toes. She went to the water's edge and stood still to watch and listen to the waves. Each wave was a glorious reminder of her being alive to enjoy this wonderful day.

The hand that touched her hand was gentle. When she turned, she saw Rebecca smiling, wrinkling her freckled nose, and wiping the blowing hair from her face.

Rebecca stood silent beside JoAnn watching the waves, and then she let go of her hand, turned, and started walking along the shoreline. She lifted up her sundress to her knees, kicked up the water spray, danced in circles, and then continued a happy skip down the beach. She took a moment to give JoAnn a goodbye wave, and then blow a kiss, before she sprinted away into the sea mist to disappear.

The End

If my gifts help even one person,
then that's who I was meant to help.

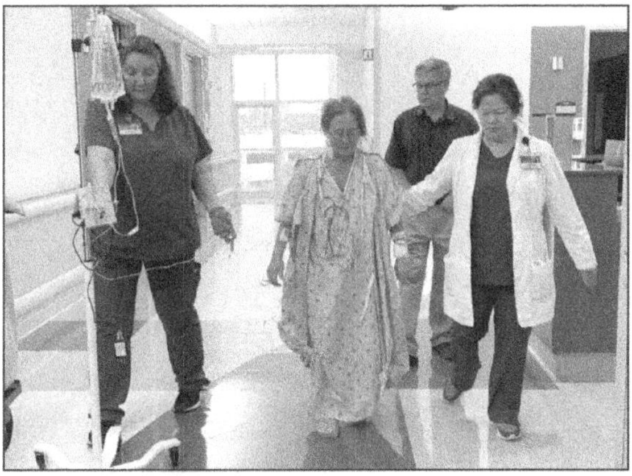

My first walk, day after surgery.

In 2014, Joan Kay was diagnosed with Autoimmune Hepatitis, a rare genetic disease that caused her body to think her liver was a foreign object and proceed to attack it until she developed cirrhosis.

On October 5, 2019, she received the gift of life, a new liver, at Mayo Clinic in Jacksonville, Florida. After her transplant she developed another autoimmune disease, Pulmonary Arterial Hypertension. She spent 60 days in ICU with heart failure. It's from her physical struggles and personal experiences that she writes the stories in this book.

Joan Kay lives in Savannah, Georgia with her husband. She is a published author of five humorous paranormal books and four Native American historical romance books.

"My gift of life has given me additional years to continue to write, paint, and enjoy my family and friends. I'm forever thankful and grateful for my donor and donor family."

On grateful wings I fly

A butterfly symbolizes acceptance of each new phase of life. To keep faith as everything around you changed.

--Lisa Kleypas

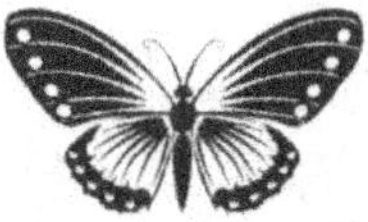

www.ingramcontent.com/pod-product-compliance
Lightning Source LLC
LaVergne TN
LVHW022311200926
848481LV00004B/1284